EVERYTHING YOU EVER WANTED TO KNOW ABOUT
PREGNANCY
BUT WERE TOO AFRAID OR EMBARRASSED TO ASK

Second Edition

BY: IDRIES J. ABDUR-RAHMAN, MD

D1114582

CONTENTS

CHAPTER 1

THE BASICS

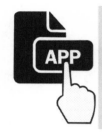 Don't forget to download the Everything Pregnancy app!

1). So, how did all of this begin?

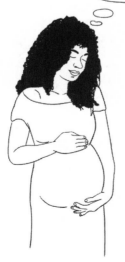

"Who knew that the birds and the bees had nothing to do with this?"

Breaking Down the Birds and the Bees:

Hopefully, your parents have already had the whole birds and bee's discussion with you. If not, take a deep breath and sit down because we might be about to blow your mind! Okay, here goes... Sometimes when a mommy loves a daddy... okay, that's enough of that. I'm pretty sure you know how this began, but let's delve a bit into the scientific nitty-gritty.

The first step in this whole sordid affair was *ovulation,* which is the process of the ovary releasing an *ovum* (egg). Once ovulation occurs, the ends of the fallopian tubes, known as the fimbria, pull the ovum into the fallopian tube where fertilization will occur.

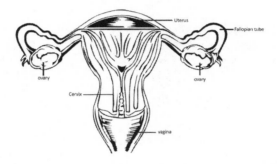

Before the ovum can be fertilized, there has to be something to actually do the fertilizing, and this is where the male of the species comes in. Hopefully, there were flowers and a nice romantic dinner involved, but regardless of how the evening started, it clearly ended with *ejaculation*, the male climax, during which millions (usually 20,000,000 or more) of little sperm are released into the vagina.

From the vagina, these little swimmers make their way through the cervix (bottom of the uterus) into the uterus and from the uterus into the fallopian tubes. And we all know who was waiting in the fallopian tubes, right? Yup, that ovum was just hanging out, waiting for a little company, and boy (or girl) did she get some. Obviously, not all pregnancies start "the old fashioned way," but regardless of whether intercourse, intrauterine insemination, or in-vitro fertilization was involved, it all ended with a sperm fertilizing an egg.

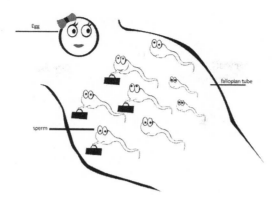

Of all the sperm that complete the long journey from the vagina to the fallopian tubes (roughly 5-10%), only one will penetrate the ovum. Once this happens, changes occur that prevent any other sperm from penetrating the egg (you can thank the zona pellucida for this) and with this, the process of making your little bundle of joy really begins.

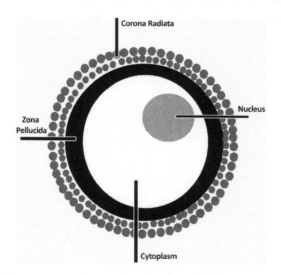

The joined sperm and ovum start the process of dividing. Remember that whole exponential growth thing from high school algebra? Well, that's what happens here as the two cells become four then sixteen and so on and so on. As this dividing ball of cells, also known as your baby, continues to divide, little hair-like projections in the fallopian tubes (called cilia) guide it down the tube and into the uterus. Once in the uterus, the dividing ball of cells attaches to and burrows into the lining of the uterus. At this point, your embryo (what your baby is called for the first eight weeks of pregnancy, beyond eight weeks it is called a fetus) starts to produce the hCG hormone that is responsible for most of the symptoms of early pregnancy and also causes that positive pregnancy test. So, there it is in a nutshell— this is how one night of passion turns into a lifetime of love (awwwwww).

2). What if I am expecting twins—how exactly did this happen?

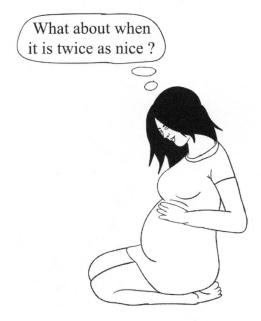

Breaking Down the Birds and the Bees and the Bees:

Well, it depends upon the type of twins that you are carrying, *identical or fraternal.*

Identical twins are genetically identical, having resulted from the same sperm and egg. At some point during the process of cellular division, the growing embryo splits into two separate embryos.

Fraternal twins, on the other hand, result from two separate sperm and two separate eggs, meaning that you likely double ovulated (once from each ovary). Genetically, fraternal twins are no more similar than any other brother or sister; they just happen to be occupying the same womb at the same time.

Identical Twins

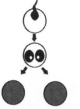

Shared Placenta

Fraternal Twins

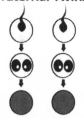

Separate Placentas

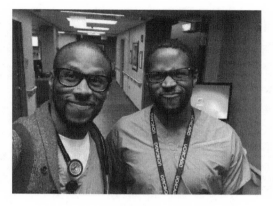

We are pretty partial to identical twins!

3). How can I be sure that I am pregnant?

"Well, all That Sweet Talking Worked. How Will I Know for Sure That I'm Pregnant?"

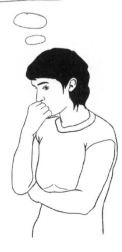

Confirming pregnancy:

There are many signs of early pregnancy, and by now you have probably become intimately acquainted with at least a few of them. Despite many subjective symptoms that indicate a likely pregnancy, there are only a few ways to actually confirm that you are pregnant.

So, what are some of the common early signs of pregnancy?

1. **Missed/Late period:** This is probably the first and most common sign that tips people off.

2. **Fatigue:** You just never seem to get enough sleep, and despite frequent naps, you feel tired all day long.

3. **Nausea with or without vomiting:** For many people, this can start as early as 3-4 weeks after fertilization and usually lasts at least through the end of the first trimester (first 14 weeks of pregnancy).

4. **Cramping and bloating:** Many women have what they often mistake for pre-menstrual symptoms.

5. **Increased vaginal discharge, often with a thick mucus:** This discharge is usually white or pale yellow and either has no odor or a very mild odor.

6. **Increased urination:** Many women feel like they are literally in the bathroom every five minutes.

7. **Breast tenderness:** This common symptom can actually be quite extreme.

8. **Headaches:** These tend to be mild but frequent, often starting mid-day.

9. **Insomnia:** Despite extreme daytime fatigue, many women find themselves tossing and turning for much of the night.

So, how can you actually confirm that you are pregnant?

1. **Urine pregnancy test:** A urine pregnancy test is the easiest and cheapest way to confirm pregnancy. Over the years, urine pregnancy tests have become more and more sensitive, and many can actually diagnose pregnancy days and sometimes even a week before a missed period.

- So, when should you take a urine pregnancy test? The Conventional wisdom is that a urine pregnancy test should be done first thing in the morning because the hCG hormone concentrates in the urine overnight. Again, with pregnancy tests becoming more and more sensitive, most tests can be taken any time of day.

- How does a urine pregnancy test work? Urine pregnancy tests detect the hCG (human chorionic gonadotropin) hormone that starts to circulate in your blood 5-7 days after fertilization. REMEMBER: A positive urine pregnancy test only means that you are pregnant; it does NOT mean that it is a normal pregnancy. While most pregnancies will be normal, more serious conditions like *ectopic pregnancies* (pregnancy that occurs outside of the uterus, usually in the fallopian tubes) will still produce a positive pregnancy test. So, it is always a good idea to contact your healthcare provider as soon as you have a positive home pregnancy test.

What about a false positive pregnancy test? There are multiple reasons for a false positive pregnancy test (a test that gives a positive result even though you are not pregnant), but thankfully, most of them are very rare. The most common cause of a false-positive test is simply letting the test sit too long after you take it. Some pregnancy tests will give a very faint false positive if they are allowed to sit too long. So, wait the 1-2 minutes that the box instructs, check the result and after that, throw the test away.

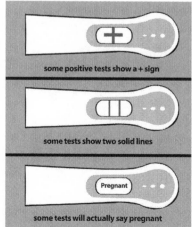

some positive tests show a + sign

some tests show two solid lines

some tests will actually say pregnant

Are there other types of pregnancy tests?

1. **Blood pregnancy test:** A blood pregnancy test also measures hCG, this time, the hCG circulating in your bloodstream. A blood test is more sensitive than a urine pregnancy test, but again, with the high sensitivity of modern urine pregnancy tests, a blood pregnancy test will only be able to diagnose pregnancy a few days before a urine test would be able to. Much like a urine pregnancy test, a positive blood pregnancy test only diagnoses a pregnancy; it cannot differentiate between a normal pregnancy and an abnormal pregnancy.

2. **Ultrasound:** An ultrasound is the only way to diagnose that you are pregnant *and* that the pregnancy is in the uterus where it belongs. Early in pregnancy, an ultrasound will likely have to be performed vaginally because that allows the sonographer (person performing the ultrasound) to get a closer look at the uterus. Every pregnancy is different, but you will usually be able to see a small embryo with a heartbeat in the uterus by about six weeks gestation (four weeks after fertilization).

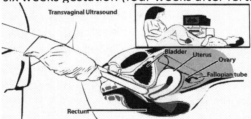

An early ultrasound is usually done through the vagina.

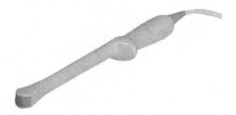

A Transvaginal ultrasound probe.

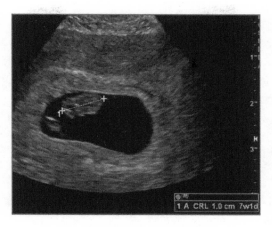

First-trimester ultrasound picture.

4). How do I determine how far along I am and when my baby is due?

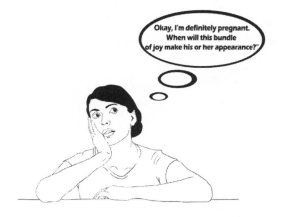

Determining Your Due Date:

Your due date will initially be determined by the first day of your last menstrual period using something called *Nagel's Rule.* To calculate your due date using Nagel's Rule you simply take the first day of the last menstrual period, add one year, subtract three months, and then add seven days. While Nagel's Rule provides a really good estimate, it is based upon an "ideal" 28-day menstrual cycle, and it assumes that you ovulate on day 14. This is not the case for many women.

♥ Ex: If your last period started on April 23rd you would add a year which takes you to April 23rd of the following year, subtract three months which takes you to January 23rd and add seven days which gives you a due date of January 30th of the following year.

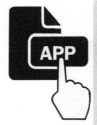

Want to figure out your due date? Head on over to the Everything Pregnancy app and check out the Nagel's Rule feature.

Now, what if you are either uncertain about when your last period started or if you have irregular periods? In this case, your provider will likely order an ultrasound to confirm your due date. Depending on how close the due date determined by your period and the due date specified by the ultrasound are, your healthcare provider will decide which date to use.

♥ REMEMBER, whatever due date your provider gives you initially (either based on your menstrual period or an early ultrasound), that is your due date. The due date does NOT change unless your provider specifically tells you that it has changed. Each subsequent ultrasound that you have will likely give you a slightly different due date. That's normal because the further along your pregnancy is, the less accurate ultrasound dating is. Just remember to always go with the earliest set due date unless your healthcare provider says otherwise.

Old Wives Tale

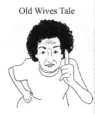

"Your due date will change throughout your pregnancy": Your due date does not change with every ultrasound. The first due date you are given is your due date unless your healthcare provider tells you otherwise.

Now that you have a due date, you are probably wondering how to determine precisely how far along you are: This is a common question and with good reason. Medical professionals usually talk weeks when dating a pregnancy, while most people talk about months. To make matters worse, when it comes to how many weeks pregnant you are, there is what is known as the gestational age and conceptional age, and these two differ by 2 weeks. So, let's break it down.

1. **Gestational Age:** Gestational age is based upon when your last period started, which for most women is about two weeks before they became pregnant. THIS is the way that medical providers will date your pregnancy. Based on this dating method, pregnancy is 40 weeks long with your due date being at the end of the 40th week.

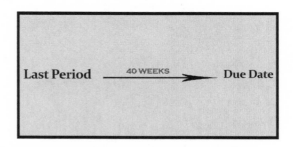

2. **Conceptional Age:** Conceptional age is based upon when you actually conceived. Using this dating method, pregnancy is 38 weeks long, and your due date is at the end of the 38th week.

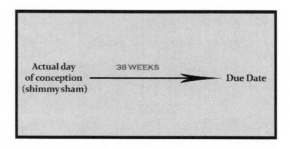

3. **Months:** Most people think of pregnancy as being nine months long, which it is. However, your due date is at the END of the 9th month, which is really the beginning of the 10th month. If you are trying to determine how many months pregnant you

are when you hear your provider refer to how many weeks pregnant you are, here is the general rule— divide the number of weeks of pregnancy by 4.5, and that will tell you how many months pregnant you are.

- ♦ Ex: If you are 30 weeks pregnant, divide 30 by 4.5, which gives you 6.7. That means that when you are 30 weeks pregnant you are basically 6 ½ months pregnant.

5). When should we tell family and friends that we are pregnant?

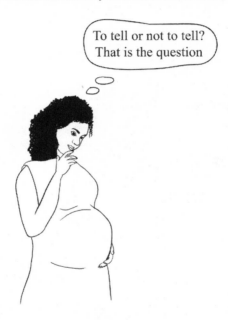

Announcing Your Pregnancy:

The short answer to that question is whenever you want to. There is no right or wrong time to share the happy news, and it is entirely up to each expectant parent/couple when they spill the beans. When it comes to sharing the news, most people are concerned that they may be telling people "too early," fearing that they may subsequently have a miscarriage.

So, when it comes to miscarriage, what is the actual risk? Well, the good news is that most recognized pregnancies will proceed normally, and the risk of miscarriage decreases as the pregnancy progresses.

- ♥ While the overall risk of miscarriage during pregnancy is approximately 50%, that includes very early pregnancies that end before they are recognized.

- ♥ By the time a pregnancy is recognized, the risk of miscarriage has already decreased to about 25%.

- ♥ By the time you have reached 7 wee ks, and ultrasound has confirmed that your pregnancy is normal and in the uterus, the risk drops to only 10%.

- ♥ By the end of the 12th week, the risk is a mere 5%.

So, the answer to when you should spill the beans is totally up to you, but those percentages should give you a little guidance in making that decision. Whatever you decide, just remember this is a happy occasion, and you should do whatever makes you feel most at ease and most comfortable.

6). When and how should we tell the children?

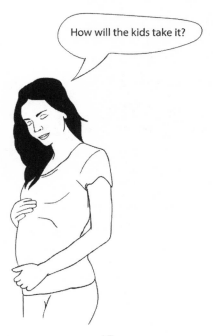

How will the kids take it?

Breaking the News to the Kiddos

Much like the question of when you should tell other family and friends, the timing of when you tell the future siblings is a personal decision. It is a question that gives many parents some trepidation, however, so here are some of the things that folks consider:

Fear of miscarriage: Any concern that you might have about having a miscarriage after telling people is no doubt magnified when it comes to telling your other children. Experiencing the sadness and disappointment of a miscarriage is difficult for adults and many parents-to-be fear that children will have even more difficulty dealing with these emotions. Just consider the age and maturity of your children. The older and more mature the child, the greater her or his ability to grasp a concept like miscarriage will likely be.

Sibling rivalry/jealousy: Probably the biggest concern of expectant non-first time mommies and daddies is sibling rivalry. The first thing to understand is that sibling rivalry is very normal, and no matter how old or mature your child is, there will always be a bit of sibling rivalry. It's normal for children to feel jealous of this unknown child who will be commanding so much of their parent's love and attention. So, what are some things that you can do to reduce the effects of sibling rivalry?

#1. Involve the children.

#2. Let the older siblings bond with the baby.

#3. Make time for the older siblings and make them feel special.

#4. Give the older siblings gifts.

Find some Big Sibling classes in your area.

1. **Stimulate early bonding.** Involve the older siblings in the process. Show them ultrasound pictures and let them talk

to the baby through your belly. Doing this will foster some of that bonding that you and your partner are already enjoying with your impending bundle of joy.

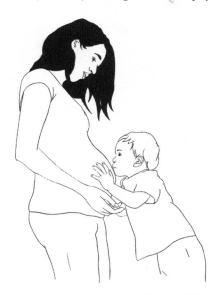

2. Involve children in baby-related activities and decisions when possible. Let them help you pick out clothes for the baby or decorate the baby's room. Once you have devised a shortlist of baby names, consider letting them have some input.

3. Spend extra time with the siblings. Their biggest fear is that you will not have time for them or that they will lose your love once the baby comes. Consider setting aside a day of the week that is just for them. This will help to ensure that they still feel like they are getting "equal time."

4. Highlight the benefits of being the big brother or sister. Hey, being the older brother or sister can have it's privileges— later bedtimes, big girl and big boy toys, etc... Make them appreciate the perks of being the older sibling.

5. Get gifts for the older siblings. The baby will definitely be lavished with all kinds of goodies from friends and family. Keep a few small gifts on hand to give to the older siblings for when the baby is getting presents.

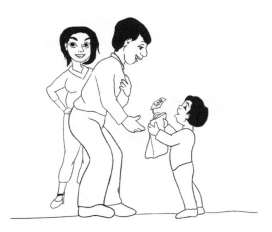

Your partner may have to take the lead on this one. Sometimes
pregnant women are just too tired or sick to be as involved as
they would like to be. This is where your partner or other close
family members can step in and pick up some of that slack.

I know they are going to spill the beans: Let's be honest here,
folks; most children (and many adults for that matter) cannot keep a
secret. Naturally, some parents-to-be are hesitant to tell soon-to-be
siblings the good news until they are ready to share that good news
with the rest of the world. Again, you know your children better
than anyone, so you are the ultimate judge. Having said that, it's
probably a good idea to wait to tell the kiddos until you are ready
for everyone else to know. Be it excitement or just the inability
to keep a secret, assume that when you share the big news with
your kids, you are sharing the big news with everyone your kids will
come into contact with.

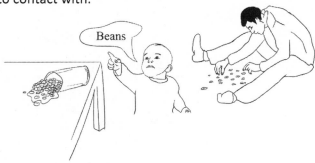

7). Should we be concerned about our pets during pregnancy?

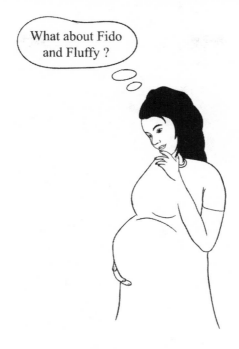

Pets and Pregnancy:

Many pet parents have concerns when it comes to the effect their new pregnancy will have on their pets and vice versa. So, what are some issues to consider?

Are pets a risk to pregnancy safety? By and large, pets do not pose a considerable risk for our mommies-to-be, but there are some exceptions to be aware of:

1. **Cats and particularly cat feces:** Cat feces can pose a serious risk to pregnant women. Cat feces may contain a parasite known as toxoplasmosis. If a pregnant woman becomes infected with toxoplasmosis, especially early in her pregnancy, it can lead to both physical malformations and severe psychological consequences for the baby. So, what should you do?

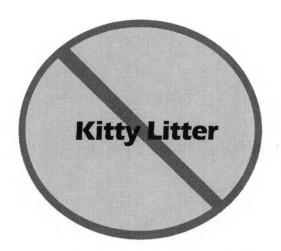

Kitty Litter

The best practice is for pregnant women to avoid kitty feces and the kitty litter box completely. I can hear all the mommies-to-be out there right now cursing their horrible luck! If this is not possible, you should wear gloves and a mask when on kitty litter duty, and you should wash your hands immediately afterward. Also, remember always to keep your cat inside; toxoplasmosis is rare in indoor cats, but outdoor cats are a different story.

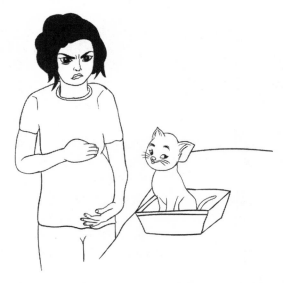

2. **Dogs:** Dogs generally pose no infection risk; just be aware of your dog's physical habits.

- If he or she is a jumper, try to break that habit to reduce the risk of them jumping onto your pregnant abdomen.

- If your dog is a biter or a nipper, try to break that habit as well before your baby arrives.

3. **Rodents like hamsters, guinea pigs, and mice:** Most rodents do pose a risk of infection. Many carry a virus known as LCMV (Lymphocytic Choriomeningitis Virus). Infections with this virus can lead to severe congenital disabilities and lead to miscarriage. So, what should you do?

   - LCMV can be contracted by coming into contact with the bodily fluids of rodents. These include feces, blood, urine, and saliva. This means avoiding bites, wearing gloves and a mask when changing cage litter, and minimizing contact with your pet during pregnancy.

4. **Reptiles**: Reptiles, including lizards and snakes, frequently carry a specific bacterium known as Salmonella. Salmonella usually causes gastrointestinal distress (nausea, vomiting, and diarrhea), but it can also lead to bacteremia (blood infection) and meningitis (infection and inflammation of the lining of the brain and spinal cord). So, what should you do?

   - It is recommended that you remove any reptiles from the home during pregnancy and especially before delivery. Infants and young children have a higher risk of contracting Salmonella infection.

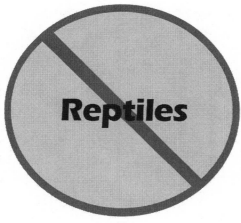

Do pets get jealous? Yes, much like human siblings-to-be, pet siblings-to-be can also experience jealousy, and it frequently is for the same reasons. Before pregnancy and delivery, pets are usually the center of attention and affection in the house. That, of course, all changes when a baby enters the equation. Much like human siblings, some things can be done to ease pet jealousy:

1. **Set aside time strictly for one-on-one interaction with your pets.** This lets them know that they are still special to you.

2. **Stock up on pet treats and toys.** Nothing says mommy and daddy still love you more than a toy or well-timed treat.

3. **Again, your partner may have to play a more active role.** This is especially true when it comes to some of the physical interactions like walks and playtime.

4. **Introduce the pet to the idea of a baby.** This can be done with the introduction of baby dolls used to teach your pet how to treat a baby.

5. **Take your pet to school.** Yes, there are actually classes to introduce your pet to the idea of a baby.

TO DO LIST

#1. Set time aside for your pet, and make him or her feel special.

#2. Give your pet toys and treats.

#3. Enroll your pet in a pet-sibling class.

TO DO LIST

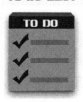

Consider finding a pet-sibling class in your area.

Are babies' safe around pets? One big area of concern for parents-to-be is the fear that their pet may harm the baby. While this is rare, you know your pet best. If your pet has shown signs of aggression, especially towards babies or children in the past, this is something that you will want to discuss with your veterinarian well before your bundle-of-joy comes. If your pet has never shown signs of aggression but you have concerns, what are some things that you can do?

1. **Introduce dolls for roleplay.** This gets your pet used to the idea of a baby and how gently they need to be handled. Make sure the doll has the same skin tone as your baby (as best as you can predict).

2. **Join a class that introduces your pet to the idea of a baby. Again, these classes actually do exist.**

3. **Expose your pet to more children (children of friends, in parks, etc.).** Obviously, exercise the greatest of care in these situations until you know how your pet will respond to little ones.

4. **Plant your baby's scent before the baby actually comes home.** Collect pieces of clothing that the baby has worn in the hospital and place them in sealed bags. Have your partner bring these bags and articles home and expose the pet to them while simultaneously rewarding him or her (giving them treats, rubbing them, etc.).

8). Are there really things that I need to avoid?

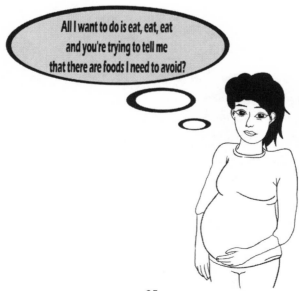

Foods and Beverages to Avoid During Pregnancy:

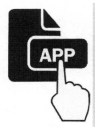

Be sure to check out the "Foods to Avoid" feature of the Everything Pregnancy app for a complete list of foods to avoid during pregnancy.

By and large, mothers-to-be are free to eat and drink anything that they can tolerate (but please keep it within your daily caloric limit), but there are a few very important exceptions. Of course, every mother-to-be is different, so be sure to discuss any dietary concerns that you have with your healthcare provider.

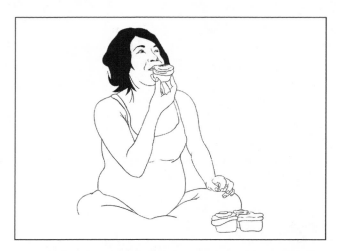

1. **Caffeine:** Caffeine does cross the placenta, but in moderation is considered safe during pregnancy. Generally, you want to limit caffeine intake to no more than 200mg per day, which is the equivalent of about 12oz total.

2. **Herbal teas:** As a general rule, you want to avoid all herbal teas unless otherwise instructed by your healthcare provider. The effects of most herbal products have not been studied during pregnancy, so their safety cannot be assured.

3. **Alcohol:** NO amount of alcohol is considered safe during pregnancy. Alcohol consumption, while pregnant, has been proven to lead to a very serious condition known as *Fetal Alcohol Syndrome (FAS)*. FAS is characterized by physical defects and severe emotional problems.

4. **Raw or undercooked meat, poultry, and fish:** Stay away from any and all raw or undercooked meats, poultry, or seafood. All of these carry a significant risk for foodborne bacteria and viruses that can have adverse effects on the pregnancy and your growing bundle of joy. So what to do?:

    ♥ Make sure that all poultry is cooked to a minimum internal temperature of 165 degrees Fahrenheit.

    ♥ Make sure that all ground meats are cooked to a minimum internal temperature of 160 degrees Fahrenheit.

    ♥ Make sure that all other meats, fish, and shellfish are cooked to a minimum internal temperature of 145 degrees Fahrenheit.

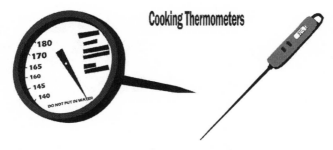

Cooking Thermometers

5. **Fish and other seafood high in mercury:** The concern with fish and seafood during pregnancy is the mercury content. Too much mercury can cause problems with your baby's neurodevelopment (brain and nerves). The good news is that there are certain fish and seafood that are lower in mercury content. So, what should you do?

    ♥ Avoid any fish or seafood high in mercury content. Generally, the larger the fish, the higher the mercury content. Seafood to avoid includes:

- ◆ Swordfish   ◆ King Mackerel
- ◆ Tilefish   ◆ Shark
- ♥ Seafood lower in mercury are not only safe during pregnancy but given their beneficial effects on baby's brain and eye development (due to the omega-3 fatty acids and protein), they are recommended (up to 12oz per week):
  - ◆ Shrimp   ◆ Anchovies
  - ◆ Trout   ◆ Catfish
  - ◆ Cod   ◆ Salmon
  - ◆ Tilapia   ◆ Pollock
  - ◆ Light canned tuna (limited to 6oz per week)

6. **Lunch/deli meats and hot dogs:** These meats can carry a high risk of listeria infection, which can lead to fetal malformations and miscarriage.

7. **Unpasteurized dairy and cheese:** All unpasteurized dairy products should be avoided, again, due to the risk of listeria infection. These unpasteurized dairy products include:
   - ♥ Soft cheeses like Roquefort, Brie, Camembert, Feta, and Gorgonzola as well as queso blanco and queso fresco.
   - ♥ Unpasteurized milk and products derived from it.

8. **Pate and other refrigerated meat spread:** These should be avoided again due to the risk of listeria.

9. **Unwashed vegetables:** Unwashed vegetables can increase the risk of toxoplasmosis infection.

10. **Raw or undercooked eggs:** Make sure all eggs also have a minimum internal temperature of 160 degrees Fahrenheit.

Old Wives Tale

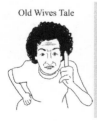

"A little wine is okay during pregnancy": An occasional glass of wine is NOT okay during pregnancy. Avoid ALL alcohol while pregnant.

TO DO LIST

Purchase a cooking thermometer and use it to test the internal temperatures of all meat and fish before consuming.

TO DO LIST

If you forget the list of foods to avoid during pregnancy, be sure to check out the "Foods to Avoid" section of the app.

CHAPTER 2

OVERVIEW OF PRENATAL CARE:
WHAT HAPPENS AND WHY?

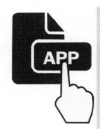

Don't forget to download the Everything Pregnancy app!

What the heck is going to happen at the first OB appointment?

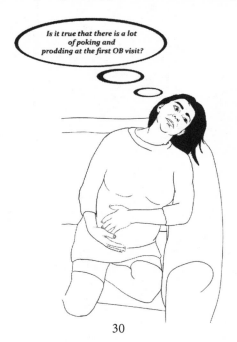

The First OB Appointment:

So, you have confirmed your pregnancy, and you have chosen a doctor or midwife, so the next big event is going to be your first OB appointment. Like most things surrounding pregnancy and delivery, this first appointment is probably the subject of lots of excitement and perhaps a little bit of apprehension as well. Fear not! The Twin Docs are going to tell you everything that you should expect from that first visit so that you sail through it like a pro! So, here is a run-down of what to expect:

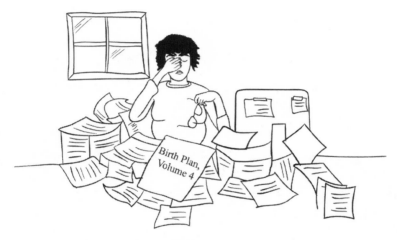

Yup, there will be a lot of paperwork!

A detailed history: When we say detailed, we mean *detailed*. Your medical provider is going to want to know everything about you and your family, right down to your shoe size. Well, maybe not your shoe size, but you get the point. Don't worry— your medical provider isn't nosey. There are actually good reasons for getting all of the information they are gathering. There are lots of things in your medical history (medical conditions, current medications, possible genetic conditions, environmental exposures) that could affect you, your pregnancy, or your baby, and the best way to predict these and prevent any potential problems is to simply ask a ton of questions. As you can imagine getting all of this information can be time-consuming, so plan at least an hour for this first visit. So, what are some things they will want to know?

1. **Prior pregnancies and outcomes:** This includes miscarriages, abortions, term, and preterm deliveries.

2. **Any medical conditions** that you have or have had in the past.

3. **Any current or past medications.**

4. **Any prior surgeries.**

5. **All vaccines received** as well as those not received.

6. **What type of work you do and where you live**: This is important to screen for potential environmental exposures.

7. **Safety concerns** (domestic violence, seatbelts, guns in the home, etc.).

8. **The presence of pets or exposure to other animals.**

9. **Your partner's personal and family medical history**, including potential genetic disorders, heart defects, or brain/spinal cord conditions.

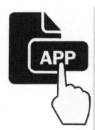

Be sure to visit the "Your History" section of the app. This has all of the information that your healthcare provider will need at your first visit. Having this information at your fingertips is important and you can save a copy to give to your healthcare provider.

Lots and lots and lots of tests: By the way, did we mention that there will be lots of lab work? Yep, much like the detailed history, these lab tests are also designed to screen for any possible conditions that could affect you, your pregnancy, or your baby. So, what tests should you expect at that first visit?

1. **A PAP smear:** Sorry to break it to you, but most medical providers will perform a PAP smear at your first OB visit if you are not current. Cervical pre-cancer and cancer are thankfully rare (because of the success of the PAP Smear), but they should definitely be screened for and what better time than during your first visit when an exam with the speculum is going to be performed anyway?

2. **Cervical cultures:** Don't take it personally, but if you are pregnant you are obviously sexually active, and the biggest risk factor for STIs (sexually transmitted infections) is, you guessed it, having sex! This isn't a judgment call on the part of your medical provider. All people are screened at the first visit because undiagnosed STIs can cause a multitude of problems, including miscarriage or preterm labor. They can also directly affect your baby after birth, and some can even cause blindness.

3. **Lots and lots of blood work:** Make sure to drink plenty of water before your first visit (and in general throughout the pregnancy) because your medical provider is going to become a vampire, drawing up to 7 tubes of blood. Again, all of these tests serve a very specific and essential purpose. So, what exactly are they checking for?

   ♦ *Blood type:* Your medical provider needs to know your blood type, and if you have specific antibodies in your blood. Certain antibodies can cross the placenta and affect your baby's wellbeing. Also, if you are a negative blood type (O-negative, AB-negative, etc.), this can cause problems in this and future pregnancies if you don't receive a shot called RhoGAM during pregnancy and again after you deliver.

   ♦ *CBC (Complete Blood Count):* Many women are anemic, and this frequently gets worse during pregnancy. If your provider diagnoses your anemia early in the pregnancy, some things can that can be done to treat it well before delivery.

   ♦ *Varicella Immunity:* Varicella is the virus that causes chickenpox. Most of us have had the chickenpox virus or the vaccine to prevent it, but sometimes our immunity to the infection wanes. Knowing your immune status is very important because if you are not immune, being exposed to the disease, especially early in pregnancy, can have some severe effects on your unborn child. The good news is that if you are not immune, your medical provider can give you a medication to prevent those effects if exposed.

33

- *Rubella Immunity:* Rubella is also known as German measles. Much like varicella most of us have been vaccinated against this, but again, immunity can wane. This infection can also cause problems for your baby if you are exposed, especially early in pregnancy.

- *HIV:* Again, not a judgment call on the part of your medical provider, but being sexually active means you are at risk for HIV infection. Treating undiagnosed HIV infection is not only crucial for mom, but it dramatically reduces the likelihood that your baby will contract the virus during pregnancy or at the time of delivery.

- *Hepatitis B and C:* Much like HIV, being sexually active puts you at higher risk for Hepatitis infection. Again, being treated early is not only good for mom, but it is also best for your baby.

- *RPR:* RPR is a test that checks for syphilis. You probably know the refrain by now, if you are sexually active you are at risk for syphilis, and much like other infections, early treatment is best for mom and baby.

- *Hemoglobin electrophoresis or Sickle Prep:* These tests check for certain conditions of the blood that can cause severe anemia in mom and potentially be transmitted to the baby. While these conditions cannot be treated, knowing your status allows the father of the baby to be tested which is important because the conditions are genetic.

- *Cystic Fibrosis Screen:* Cystic fibrosis is a genetic condition that can cause a multitude of problems for your baby, including intestinal issues and lung problems. Parents can be carriers of this disease even though they have no symptoms, which is why screening is so important.

- *Specialized Carrier and Condition Screening:* Depending on your ethnicity, your provider may perform other specific genetic screening tests. Be sure to ask her or him if other testing is required or recommended.

Determine your due date: One of the first things that your medical provider will do is determine when your baby is due. There are a few ways to do this (have we said do and due enough yet?)

1. **Nagel's Rule:** If you are certain of when your last period started and how often your periods normally come, your medical provider can determine your due date with pretty precise accuracy just by using a bit of simple math. Nagel's Rule states that you take the first day of your last normal period, add a year, subtract three months, and then add seven days. It's just that simple. If your periods are irregular, this method isn't as accurate, but it still provides a decent estimate.

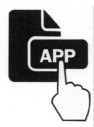

Check out the Due Date Calculator to determine your approximate due date.

2. **Ultrasound:** If you are uncertain of when your last period started or if your periods are irregular, your provider will likely order an ultrasound to determine how many weeks pregnant you are and what your due date will be. The earlier the ultrasound, the better in terms of its accuracy.

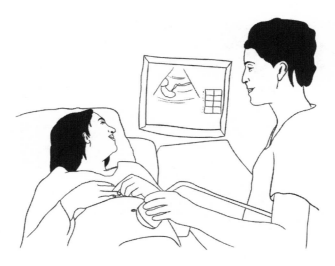

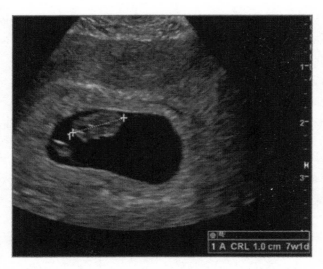

Your baby's first picture will probably look more like this.

3. **Pelvic examination:** A simple pelvic exam will allow your provider to determine how large your uterus is, which corresponds roughly to how far along your pregnancy is. This will also allow him or her to evaluate the bones of your pelvis. Knowing the shape of your pelvic bones is essential when it comes time for delivery.

Prescription for Prenatal vitamins and other medications:

1. **Prenatal Vitamins:** You may have already started taking an over-the-counter prenatal vitamin. If you have not, your provider will likely prescribe a prenatal vitamin for you.

2. **DHA/Omega-3 Fatty Acids:** Many prenatal vitamins come with supplemental DHA/Omega-3 fatty acids. If your vitamin does not come with this supplement, consider purchasing it separately over-the-counter. DHA/Omega-3 fatty acids play an important role in your baby's neurodevelopment (brain development) and the development of good eyesight.

3. **Depending upon your medical history, your medical provider may prescribe other medications for you.** Make sure to

discuss any medications that you are currently taking with your provider to determine which are appropriate to continue and which may need to be stopped or substituted

TO DO LIST

Consider taking your prenatal vitamin before bed with a light snack. The iron in prenatal vitamins helps prevent or treat anemia but it can also make your nausea worse.

TO DO LIST

If you are still experiencing stomach irritation or if your prenatal vitamin is causing constipation, speak with your provider about a low or no-iron formulation.

TO DO LIST

No excuses! If you have problems swallowing pills, gummy prenatal vitamins are a great option.

Discuss your pregnancy-related fears, concerns, and expectations: You and your medical provider will likely become almost like BFFs over the next nine months and beyond. It is crucial that you feel comfortable talking to your provider, and a big part of this is discussing any fears and concerns that you have. Trust me, no matter the question, your provider has likely heard it at least a hundred times before! Your provider will probably also discuss a brief outline of what to expect during the course of your pregnancy, prenatal care as well as the post-partum period (though this part may come later in the pregnancy). Again, ask any questions that you might have. It's is all in a day's work for your medical provider, but for you, this is a once in a lifetime event with many unknowns. Questions should always be welcome.

What happens during my first-trimester office visits?

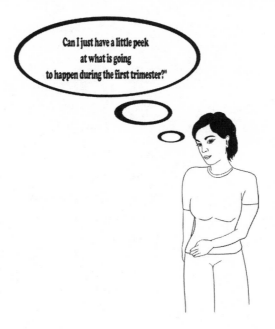

First Trimester Prenatal Care:

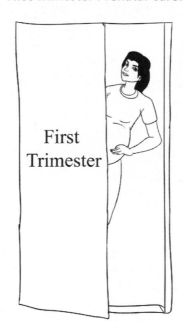

For many women, the first trimester of pregnancy is a time filled with lots of excitement, lots of nerves, and lots of nausea. Of the three trimesters, the first trimester is probably the least favorite for most women because they experience all of the not so fun parts of pregnancy (sore breasts, fatigue, nausea, vomiting, constipation, etc.) and none of the fun parts (feeling the baby move, people fawning over your pregnant belly, knowing the baby's gender). Just remember the wise advice somebody gave to that poor kitty on the poster: Hang in There Baby, because it will get better.

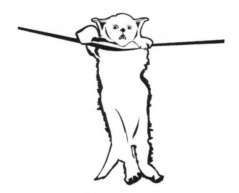

What is the first trimester? The first trimester is the first one-third of the pregnancy. It starts with the first day of your last menstrual period (so obviously before you were even pregnant, and definitely before you knew you were pregnant, unless of course, you are clairvoyant) and goes through the 14th week of your pregnancy. Some folks also think of it as the first three months of your pregnancy, whatever floats your boat.

What can I expect during prenatal care in the first trimester? Well, we already talked all about your first prenatal care visit, so let's highlight some of what you can expect after all the poking and probing of that first visit:

1. **Genetic Testing**: Testing for Down's Syndrome and other genetic disorders is one of most significant areas of concerns for many parents-to-be. Should you test or should you not? What happens if a potential problem is discovered? Let's start by saying that genetic testing is ALWAYS optional but generally

recommended. When it comes to genetic testing most people fall into one of three camps: The *"we want to know because if there is an issue we would consider terminating the pregnancy"* camp, the *"we don't want to know anything because it will only make us nervous"* camp and the largest camp, *"we want to know about the possibilities for informational and preparation purposes"*. In most cases, we usually recommend genetic testing because it allows for parental preparation while also allowing your medical team to prepare for possible issues or complications that might arise. So, having said that, what are your options?

- *CVS: CVS or chorionic villi sampling* is a procedure that uses a needle to remove chorionic villi from the placenta. Chorionic villi are early placental cells that contain your baby's genetic information.

  - This test can be used to screen for a multitude of genetic conditions including Down syndrome and cystic fibrosis.

  - It is generally performed between 9-13 weeks of pregnancy and must be performed by a specialist.

  - It is associated with a 1-2% risk of miscarriage.

- *NT/First-trimester screen:* NT or Nuchal Translucency is a targeted ultrasound that measures the thickness of the back of the baby's neck. In certain genetic conditions, this area can be thicker than usual. This ultrasound is usually combined with a special blood test that measures the levels of certain hormones in mom's blood; these can also be abnormal when certain fetal medical conditions exist.

  - It is generally performed between 10-12 weeks of pregnancy.

  - It does not increase the risk of miscarriage, does not require a specialist, and can often be performed in your provider's office.

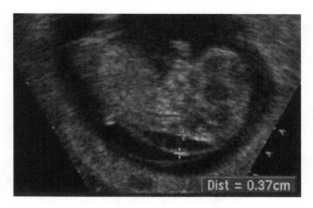

Ultrasound measuring the nuchal translucency (NT)

- ◆ *NIPT with AFP:* NIPT, or Non-Invasive Prenatal Testing, is a newer technique that extracts fragments of your baby's cells that normally circulate in mom's blood. This is combined with a second blood test looking specifically for AFP (Alpha-Fetoprotein), a hormone that can be elevated when babies have neural tube (the structure that produces the brain and spinal cord) defects like spina bifida.

  - ○ NIPT blood testing can be performed from 10 weeks onward. The AFP blood test is drawn at or after 15 weeks.

  - ○ This does not require a specialist and can be performed in your provider's office.

2. **Hearing your baby's heartbeat for the first time:** If you have an ultrasound performed during the first trimester, you will likely see and hear the baby's heartbeat. Additionally, your provider will use a device called a Doppler to listen to the baby's heartbeat at every visit, starting at about 10-12 weeks of pregnancy. DON'T be alarmed if your provider cannot find the heartbeat right away with the doppler. Many factors come into play, including your weight, the position of your uterus, and the baby's location within the uterus at the time that your medical provider is trying to find the heartbeat.

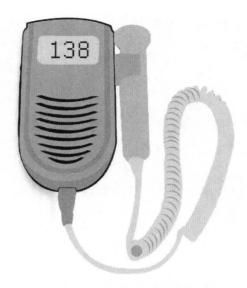

Doppler used to measure fetal heart rate.

3. **Monitoring your weight:** The topic of weight gain during pregnancy is one that many women hate to think about or discuss, but it really shouldn't be. Let's just establish the fact that weight gain is not only natural and normal during pregnancy, but it is actually a GOOD thing. If you are gaining weight, that means your baby is gaining weight. The key is to make sure that your weight gain is healthy. So, what exactly is normal during the first trimester? Well, many women don't actually gain weight, and depending upon the severity of morning sickness, some may lose a bit of weight during the first trimester. For those that do gain weight, it is generally limited to a couple of pounds, and yes, your provider will be checking your weight at every visit so be prepared.

4. **Monitoring your urine:** As if having your weight checked at every visit isn't enough, you will also have to master the fine art of peeing in a tiny cup before this joyous journey is complete. And if you think that is difficult now, just wait until you have a bowling ball blocking your view! There is a good reason for checking your urine, however. Your provider will be checking for signs of a UTI (urinary tract infection), which is

more common during pregnancy and left untreated, can lead to serious complications for mom and baby. They will also be checking your urine for something called ketones which let us know if you are hydrating enough, as well as checking for glucose or sugar, which in excessive amounts could be a sign of diabetes, and protein, which can be an early sign of a condition called pre-eclampsia.

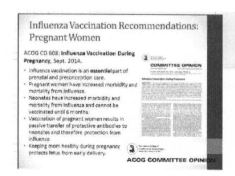

5. **Flu Vaccine:** ACOG, the American College of Obstetricians and Gynecologists and RCOG, the Royal College of Obstetricians and Gynecologists (UK), both recommend that all pregnant women get a flu vaccine if they will be pregnant during any part of flu season. Flu season is from October through May, so that means every woman will be pregnant during some part of flu season. When it comes to timing, the earlier, the better as flu during pregnancy can have some grave consequences for mom and baby, including an increased risk of death.

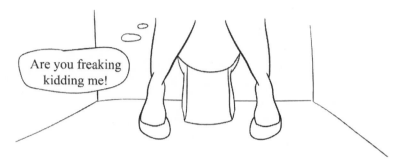

What happens during my second-trimester office visits?

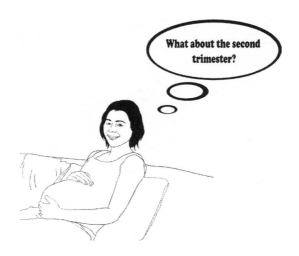

Second Trimester Prenatal Care:

Yay, you! You have survived the first trimester, and you are now entering what many people consider to be the Golden Period of pregnancy. The ills of the first trimester are by and large gone; you are starting to look pregnant and feel the baby move for the first time, and the discomforts of the third trimester are yet to come. So, like Virginia Slims once said, you've come a long way baby. Enjoy this time!

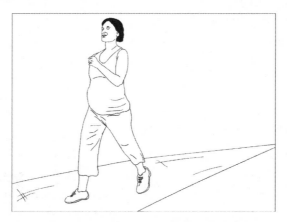

Unlike Virginia Slims, we don't want to see you smoking!

What is the second trimester? The second trimester starts at 14 weeks and goes through 28 weeks of pregnancy. Put another way, the fourth, fifth, and sixth months of pregnancy are the second trimester.

What can I expect in terms of prenatal care during the second trimester?
Prenatal care during the second trimester is when stuff really starts to get good. You are regularly hearing the baby's heartbeat, and if you want to know, this is when most folks will find out the baby's gender.

1. **Genetic Testing:** There are a multitude of tests to screen for genetic disorders like Down's Syndrome including the first trimester options of CVS, nuchal translucency/first-trimester screen and NIPT testing with AFP, all of which were outlined earlier. The trend is moving towards earlier and earlier genetic testing; there are some options that can be done during the early weeks of the second-trimester as well. Second- trimester screening options include:

   ◆ *Quad Screen or Penta Screen:* A blood test that screens for specific chromosomal abnormalities like Down syndrome as well as neural tube defects (brain and spinal cord malformations) by measuring the levels of certain hormones circulating in mom's bloodstream.

     ○ This test can only be performed in the second trimester, usually between 15-20 weeks of pregnancy.

     ○ It does not require a specialist and can be performed in your provider's office with a simple blood draw.

   ◆ *Amniocentesis:* This is a test that uses a needle to withdraw a small amount of the amniotic fluid from your uterus. Amniotic fluid contains fetal cells that can be evaluated for chromosomal issues and a wide array of genetic disorders.

     ○ This test is usually performed between 16-20 weeks' gestation but can be done at any time up to delivery.

     ○ There is an approximately 0.5% risk of pregnancy loss, and it can be performed by a specialist or a general OB/ GYN.

   ◆ *Level two ultrasound:* An ultrasound that is performed by a specialist that takes a more detailed look at your baby's anatomy and specifically at organs that are more likely to be abnormal in babies with certain genetic or medical conditions.

○ This test is generally performed at about 20 weeks of pregnancy.

○ It is non-invasive but usually requires a specialist.

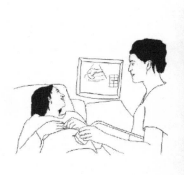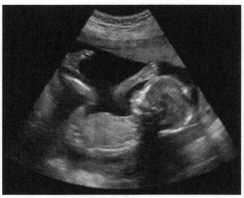

By now, your baby will be looking more like a baby.

2. **Anatomy Ultrasound:** Without a doubt, the anatomical ultrasound is the star of the prenatal care show for most parents-to-be. It is the first time that you will get a detailed look at your baby including her or his facial features, and it may be the first time that you will learn if she is a she or he is a he. This exam usually takes about 30 minutes, and it evaluates the baby's major organs including the brain and spinal cord, the heart, the kidneys and bladder, the upper and lower limbs, and of course the gender. This will likely come as no surprise to most folks, but sometimes babies aren't cooperative. This might mean that the ultrasonographer cannot determine the sex or that they cannot get all of the necessary views to evaluate the organs. In the case of the latter, you will likely have another ultrasound in 4-6 weeks to take another look. In the case of the former, you might just have to wait until that big moment in the delivery room when your doctor or midwife yells out the three words you've been waiting for, "it's a ...."

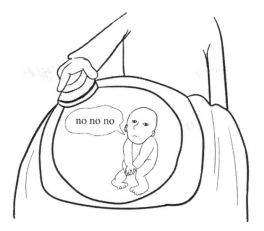

3. **Diabetes Screening:** Most folks don't know it, but the hormones of pregnancy can increase a woman's chance of developing diabetes. Thankfully for most this is strictly confined to pregnancy, hence the name gestational diabetes. For others, however, they may have had diabetes before pregnancy, and the diagnosis is just delayed for lack of previous testing. So, what exactly does this test involve?

♦ *1-hour glucose test:* This is the most common test performed to check for diabetes. It requires our mommy-to-be to drink a sugary drink called Glucola and have her blood tested one hour later to check the glucose (sugar) level. If your glucose level is below the threshold, all is well. If it is above the threshold (130-140 depending upon your medical provider), you will have to take a 3-hour test (see below) for confirmation.

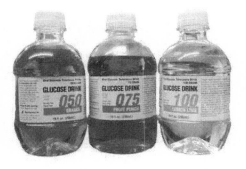

Different Glucola glucose drinks.

- *2-hour glucose test:* Instead of a one-hour test (and a three-hour test if your one-hour test is too high), some providers will perform a two-hour test. Much like the one-hour test, the two-hour test requires our mommy-to-be to drink a sugary Glucola drink (this time with a bit more glucose in it) and have her blood drawn three times-before the drink, one hour after, and two hours after finishing the drink. For this test, you have to fast for 12 hours beforehand. The upside is that it is a one-step test. This means that if you pass you pass and if you don't pass, no further testing is necessary.

- *3-hour glucose test:* Well, if there is a one hour test and a two-hour test, you probably guessed that there had to be a three-hour test as well, right? The three-hour test is performed when your one-hour test was above the threshold. Much like the two-hour test, the three-hour test requires a 12-hour fast beforehand. You are given an even higher dose of the Glucola drink, and your blood is drawn four times (before you drink, then 1, 2, and 3 hours after finishing the drink). Two or more abnormal values are indicative of gestational diabetes.

4. **Monitoring your fundal height:** The fundal height is the distance from the top of your pubic bone to the top of the uterus (known as the fundus). Most medical providers will start checking the fundal height at about 18-20 weeks of pregnancy. Your fundal height in centimeters should roughly equal how many weeks pregnant you are plus or minus two centimeters. This measurement gives your provider a quick way to monitor your baby's growth and your amniotic fluid levels.

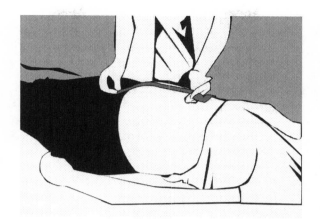

5. **Monitoring your weight and urine:** I hate to break it to you, but the weight and urine monitoring will continue. How much weight you should gain during the second and third trimesters depends upon your BMI (Body Mass Index) at the start of pregnancy and other factors, including the number of babies you are carrying. We discuss normal weight gain during pregnancy in much more detail in CHAPTER 19 entitled, wait for it…. "Weight Gain".

What happens during my third-trimester office visits?

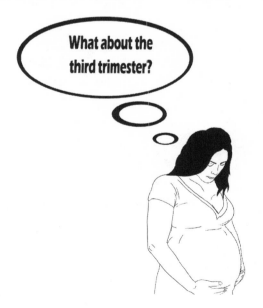

What about the third trimester?

Third Trimester Prenatal Care

Now it's time to celebrate! You are rounding the bend; you are getting closer to that finish line, and you can definitely see the light at the end of the tunnel. You are in the third trimester, and your time as a mother-to-be is coming to an end!

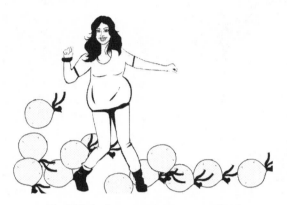

The Third trimester means party time!

What is the third trimester? The third trimester goes from 28 weeks through the end of pregnancy. The third trimester is the seventh, eighth, and ninth months of your pregnancy.

What can I expect in terms of prenatal care during the third trimester? By now you have this whole prenatal care thing down, and you have a pretty good idea of what to expect at your visits. The biggest change during the third trimester is that your visits will become more frequent, going from every four weeks to every three weeks, then every two weeks, and in the last month of your pregnancy every week. Like all of your other visits, you will still be regularly hearing the baby's heartbeat, having your uterine size (fundal height) checked, and having your blood pressure and urine monitored. Here are some of the new things that you can expect during the third trimester:

1. **RhoGAM shot:** Your blood type was checked at your first prenatal visit, and many people probably know if they are blood type A, B, AB or O. What you may not know is if you are a positive or negative blood type. Most folks are positive, but roughly 15% of us are negative (A-, B-, AB-, or O-). If you

are a negative blood type you will need the RhoGAM shot. RhoGAM prevents a condition called *alloimmunization* in which the baby's blood mixes with mom's blood causing mom's body to produce antibodies to baby's blood. These antibodies primarily cause issues in subsequent pregnancies, but if they are produced early enough, they can cause problems during your current pregnancy as well. The RhoGAM shot is given at 28 weeks and again after delivery if your baby is confirmed to have a positive blood type (A+, B+, AB+, or O+). If you have an accident or some type of trauma at any point during the pregnancy, you should have a RhoGAM shot if you have a negative blood type even if you already received a dose.

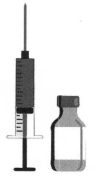

Rho(D) Immune Globulin (Human) RhoGAM®

Ultra-Filtered PLUS – 300 µg Dose (1500 IU*)
Thimerosal-Free
*International Units

Caution: RhoGAM should be administered to the unsensitized Rh-negative woman preferably within three days after miscarriage or delivery of an Rh-positive infant. **DO NOT INJECT INFANT.**
Rx Only
For Intramuscular Use Only—Do Not Inject Intravenously
The patient and physician should discuss the risks and benefits of this product.

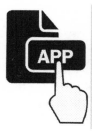

If you haven't yet, be sure to visit the "Your History" section to fill out all of your important medical and health information including your blood type. Having this information at your fingertips can be very important.

2. **Tdap vaccine:** The Tdap vaccine (tetanus, diphtheria, and acellular pertussis) is recommended for all pregnant women during their third trimester of pregnancy. Pertussis, also known as whooping cough, can cause acute respiratory distress in infants and in some cases, even lead to death. Being vaccinated will prevent you from contracting and passing the illness on to your baby while also allowing the antibodies that you produce after vaccination to cross the placenta and give your baby temporary protection after delivery. Don't worry; your partner hasn't gotten away clean on this one— it is also recommended that any adult who will be in close proximity to the baby (siblings, dad, caregivers) should also be vaccinated with the Tdap vaccine.

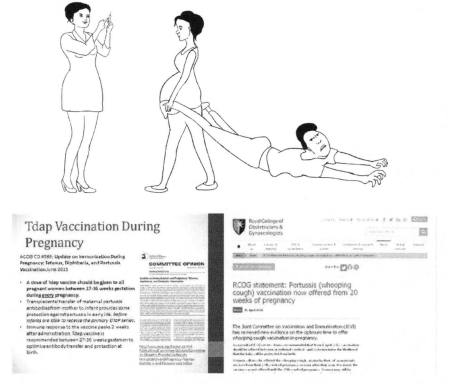

3. **Group B Strep testing:** Group B Strep (GBS) is a bacterium that we all have in our GI (gastrointestinal) tracts. This bacterium

at times, however, can also be found in the vagina (20-30% of women). At 36 weeks of pregnancy, a quick swab will be placed in the vagina and swabbed over the perineum (the area between the vagina and anus) to test for the presence of this bacteria. If you are found to be positive for GBS, you will be given IV antibiotics during labor to prevent transmitting the bacteria to your baby during delivery. Babies who contract GBS during delivery are at risk for blood infections (sepsis), brain and spinal cord infections (meningitis), respiratory infections, and even death. Being positive for GBS in one pregnancy does not mean that you will inevitably be positive in subsequent pregnancies, so you will be re-tested with each pregnancy.

4. **Pelvic/Cervical exams:** Most women will have at least one pelvic examination during the last month of pregnancy. The frequency of exams will depend upon your provider's preference and your medical history. The purpose of the pelvic exam is to determine if your cervix (the bottom of your uterus) has started to dilate (open), efface (thin out), and soften, all of which are signs that labor may be coming soon or may have already started. The pelvic exam also allows your provider to make sure that your baby is in the right position (head down) and to see how low or high in the birth canal your baby's head is.

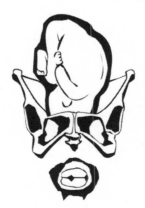

5. **Third-trimester ultrasound:** Some providers will routinely do an ultrasound during the third trimester to get a guesstimate of your baby's weight, to monitor your amniotic fluid levels, and

to check the baby's position. Again, this is at your provider's discretion, and not all providers do an ultrasound in the third trimester in the absence of a particular concern.

5). What happens during office visits if I'm past my due date?

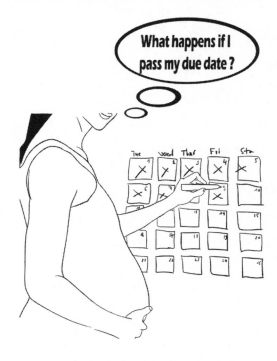

Prenatal Care Beyond Your Due Date:

Okay, we hear ya. It's been a fun or at least an interesting party, but the party is over and you are most definitely ready to call it quits. Your dream of having that baby a week or so early, or at least on your due date, has been dashed and much to your chagrin, you are still pregnant even though your "due date" has come and gone.

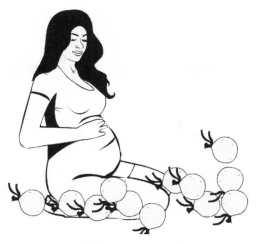

Oppppsss, guess the party is over!

What is post-dates, and how does it differ from post-due dates? Believe it or not, there is a difference between being post-due date and post-dates. Post-due date means that you have passed your due date. Post-dates means that you have made it to or past 41 weeks (which is a week or more past your due date). Interesting factoid for dinner parties, but at the end of the day you are still pregnant, and you are wondering when things are going to get started!

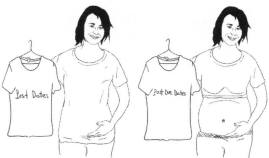

What can I expect in terms of prenatal care past my due date? If you are past your due date and your little bundle of joy is still hanging out in there don't worry, you are not alone. Only 5% of women actually deliver on their due date, and first babies do tend to go past their due date. Remember, your due date is not exact; it is just an estimation, and it is influenced by how certain you were about the date of your last period and how early your first ultrasound was. Sometimes, this estimate can be off by up to a couple of weeks. The vast majority of post-due date and post-date pregnancies go off without a hitch, but there are some potential risks to pregnancies that extend beyond their due date. These include low amniotic fluid level, meconium (when the baby defecates in the amniotic fluid), reduced placental function, and while rare, stillbirth does become more common. This is why many providers will monitor women more closely once their pregnancy has extended past the due date.

1. **More frequent visits:** Some providers will start to see you twice weekly once you have passed your due date, and almost all providers will if you go past 41 weeks.

2. **Testing to monitor for fetal well-being:** Because of the small but increased potential for complications after passing your due date, most providers will do things to ensure that your baby is still doing well in utero including:

   ♦ A). Kick Counts: These are quick and easy and can be done almost anywhere. Ideally, mom should sit or lie in a quiet place and simply count how many times the baby moves over a specified period of time. Different providers have different preferences in terms of what that period of time is, so be sure to ask your provider what she or he recommends. We recommend that you should feel 10 or more movements over an hour. Sometimes a little caffeine or sugar will perk baby up if necessary. If you get less then 10 movements over an hour, we recommend starting the count over and trying for another hour. If you still get less than 10 movements over that second hour, we recommend that you go to your hospital or birthing center for further evaluation.

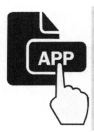

The "Kick Counts" section of the app should become your best friend during the third trimester. You can use this feature to easily time and record your kick counts.

If you are ever concerned that your baby is not moving as much as usual, be sure to do kick counts.

♦ B). Ultrasound for AFI: AFI stands for amniotic fluid index, and this is a measurement of how much amniotic fluid is in your uterus. One of the first signs that the placenta is not working optimally is the production of less amniotic fluid. Adequate levels of amniotic fluid are a good indicator that your baby is doing just fine.

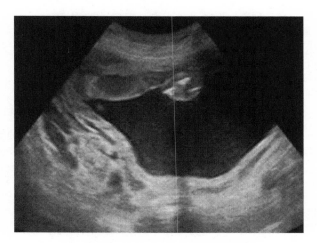

Ultrasound showing amniotic fluid (black).

♦ C). Non-stress tests: NST for short, this is a test that can be done in the hospital, birth center, or office setting. It involves placing one monitor on your belly to detect the fetal heart rate and a second monitor to detect contractions. It usually takes no more than 20 minutes, and if there is adequate fluctuation in the baby's heart rate (what we call reactivity), the testing is considered reassuring. This test may be done once weekly or twice weekly depending upon your provider's preference.

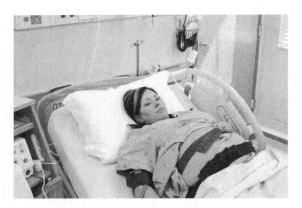

NST (Non-stress test) monitoring.

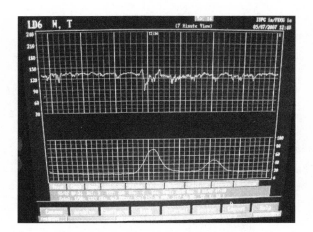

NST tracing.

♦   D). Biophysical Profile: BPP for short, is an NST and an
    ultrasound looking at four things; the amniotic fluid level
    (AFI), the frequency of baby's movements, the baby's tone
    (if the baby is flexing and extending his or her arms and
    legs), and the frequency of baby's practice breathing
    (remember, babies don't actually breathe inside of the
    uterus). A BPP is scored on a scale of 10 (2 points for each
    of the five parameters). If your baby scores an 8 or 10 on
    his or her BPP, you can rest comfortably that all will likely
    be well.

Is there anything that I can do to stimulate labor? There are tons of old wives' tales out there telling you what you can do to induce labor. Most of them are called old wives' tales for a reason and will do nothing more than potentially make you uncomfortable. Worry not! The Twin Docs are here to share some scientifically proven things that may actually induce labor! Here is a list, BUT as always discuss these with your provider before attempting them, and NEVER try them before your 39th week of pregnancy:

1. **Nipple stimulation:** Stimulating the nipples causes your brain to release the hormone oxytocin. Oxytocin is the primary hormone responsible for labor, and many healthcare providers use a synthetic form of it, called Pitocin when inducing labor.

2. **Sex:** For many women, it is sex that got you here in the first place, and it might just be sex that ends this journey for you as well. Semen has a substance in it known as *prostaglandins*; these chemicals soften the cervix and potentially stimulate cervical thinning and dilation, which can induce labor.

3. **Evening primrose oil:** This can be taken either orally or vaginally. It has a substance in it called *linoleic acid* that stimulates your body to release prostaglandins, which again can cause your cervix to dilate and thin out possibly inducing labor. Speak with your provider before inserting anything into your vagina.

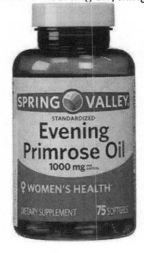

4. **Acupuncture and Acupressure:** There are specific pressure points in the feet, ankles, lower back, and hands that are believed to stimulate labor.

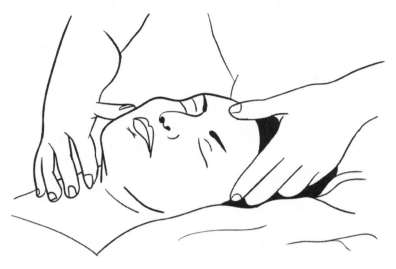

Acupressure

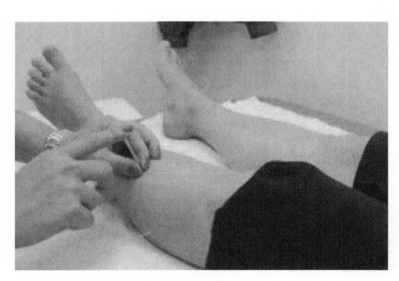

Acupuncture.

5. **Red raspberry leaf tea:** This is also said to stimulate uterine contractions, which can possibly induce labor.

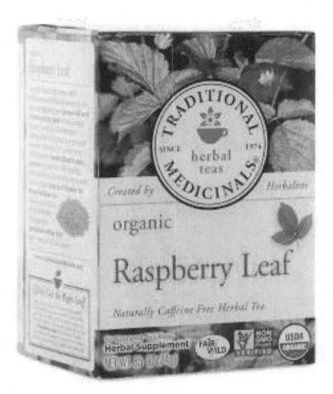

When should we consider inducing labor? There are a lot of clinical considerations that need to be taken into account when it comes to inducing labor, so ultimately, this is a discussion that you need to have with your healthcare provider. Most providers will have a cut-off date beyond which they usually will not let pregnancy progress. For most physicians and some midwives that cut off is 41 weeks, while others may let a pregnancy go to 42 weeks. Our practice is that we recommend labor induction by 41 weeks because of the increased risk of maternal and fetal complications that can occur after 41 weeks, including stillbirth.

CHAPTER 3

SKIN

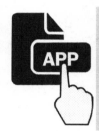

Don't forget to download the Everything Pregnancy app!

1). Does your skin really get darker during pregnancy?

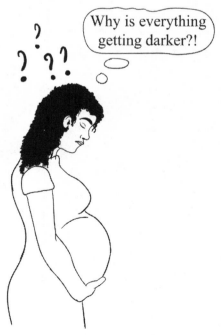

Why is everything getting darker?!

Skin Darkening During Pregnancy:

Is this real, or am I imagining this? This is one of the most common complaints that we hear from patients, so don't fret because this is totally normal.

Why is it happening? Part of the hCG hormone that you produce during pregnancy is very similar to another hormone called MSH or melanocyte-stimulating hormone. This hormone is responsible for skin pigmentation. The end result is that the rising hCG levels cause your pigment-producing cells to go into overdrive.

Old Wives Tale

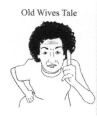

"Your skin is getting darker because it is dirty": *Skin darkening during pregnancy has nothing to do with hygiene and scrubbing it will not make it to go away.*

Tell me more: Just about any part of the body can become darker, but some of the most common areas include the face (called melasma), the breasts and nipples, the genitals, and the line that runs down the middle of your growing belly (known as the *linea nigra*). Also, any skin that is exposed to sun or friction can become more easily discolored.

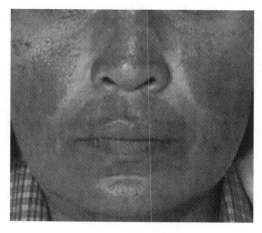

Patient with melasma.

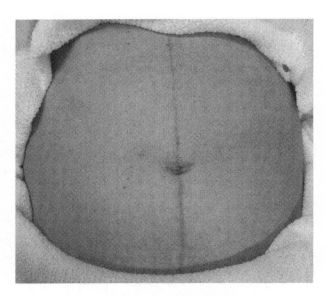

Typical linea nigra of pregnancy.

Can I treat this? *While this can't be prevented (because it is related to normal hormone production during pregnancy), there are things that you can do to reduce the effect.*

1). **Sun protection:** Sun protection is always important, and it plays a definite role here. Wear an spf-50 or higher sunscreen, reapply it frequently, and be sure to cover sun-exposed areas with clothing whenever possible.

2). **Use hypoallergenic or fragrance-free products:** We are talking lotions, soaps, detergents, etc. Anything that you either apply directly to your skin or apply to things that then touch your skin should be hypoallergenic and fragrance free.

Will this get better? Absolutely! Like most pregnancy-related conditions caused by hormones, once the pregnancy ends and the hormones go away, so does the condition.

When should I call my provider? If you notice an area of discoloration that grows rapidly, has irregular borders, is raised, or causes pain or discomfort you should inform your provider.

2). Do pregnancy and dry skin go together like peas and carrots?

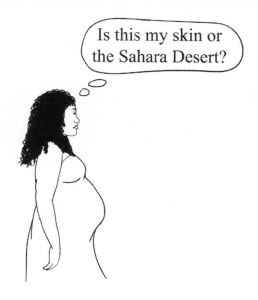

Dry Skin and Pregnancy:

Is this real, or am I imagining this? Once again, you are not imagining this. Dry skin during pregnancy is a very real and common complaint.

Why is this happening? It's a constant refrain during pregnancy and this book, but you can in large part blame it on the hormones. Inadequate hydration also can produce dry skin during pregnancy, so make sure you are chugging that water because you can't blame the hormones for everything!

Tell me more: Hormonal elevations during pregnancy reduce the elasticity and overall moisture content of the skin. Combine this with the relative dehydration that occurs as more of your body's fluids are shifted to the growing uterus and baby, and your skin can end up a dry, flakey mess! Many pregnant women, especially in the first trimester of pregnancy, have a difficult time adequately hydrating because of nausea or morning sickness, which only worsens the problem.

Can I treat this? The hormonal part of the picture can't be fixed, but there are things that you can do to improve dry skin:

1). **Hydrate, hydrate, hydrate:** Hydration is vital during pregnancy for a multitude of reasons, and helping to combat dry skin is just one of them.

2). **Humidify:** Having a humidifier in your bedroom will increase the moisture content of the air, which will, in turn, increase your skin's moisture content.

3). **Moisturize, moisturize, moisturize:** Using a moisturizer that is rich in emollients is like external hydration for your skin, and it will definitely relieve the intense itch associated with dry skin.

TO DO LIST

#1). Hydrate

#2). Get a humidifier

#3). Use lots of moisturize.

Will this get better? It sure will! The hormonal effect on the skin will resolve as the hormone levels return to normal in the 6-12 weeks after delivery.

When should I call my provider? If you notice plaques (raised, sometimes scaly areas) on the skin or discoloration let your provider know.

3). Why do I feel like one big rash?

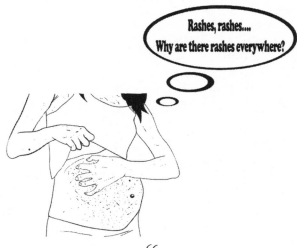

Rashes and Itching During Pregnancy:

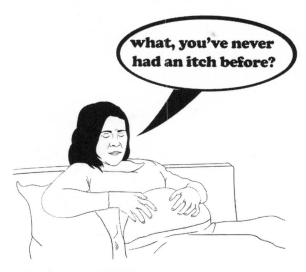

Is this real, or am I imagining this? Rashes during pregnancy are very common.

Why is it happening? The *why* depends upon the *what*, but like most changes during pregnancy, hormonal fluctuations are largely to blame. We already talked about the normal increase in skin pigmentation and sensitivity that occurs during pregnancy, so it makes sense that from time to time rashes might pop up. A rash, after all, is just an itchy area of increased skin pigmentation.

Tell me more: The three most common rashes during pregnancy are:

1). **PUPPS:** Which is an acronym for *pruritic urticarial papules and plaques of pregnancy,* is the most common pregnancy-associated rash, occurring in up to 1% of all pregnancies.

   ♦ PUPPS tends to occur more during first pregnancies (especially with male fetuses— those dang boys!), and it usually develops during the third trimester (and frequently the last month of pregnancy).

   ♦ PUPPS is characterized by an intensely itchy, red rash that starts on the belly and eventually spreads to the extremities.

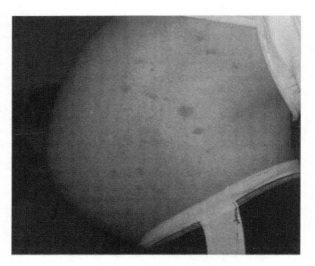

Typical PUPPS rash.

2). **Striae (stretch marks):** These aren't really rashes, but they are the most common skin change noted in pregnancy, and since they frequently cause itching, we decided to include them here. Hate to break it to you, but despite common misconception, moisturizers and cocoa butter will not prevent stretch marks from forming. Moreover, while we are bursting bubbles, here is some more "good" news for you— while most people think that stretch marks only occur on the belly, they are frequently also found on the arms and legs.

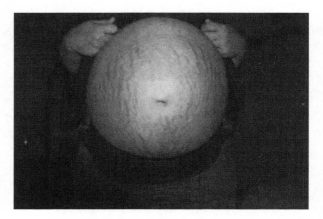

Stretch marks can be red or purple.

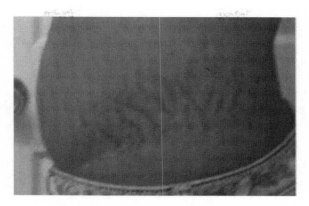

Stretch marks can be darker in darker-skinned people.

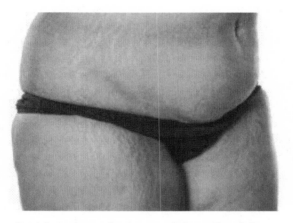

Stretch marks tend to become lighter after delivery.

3). **Cholestasis:** Is the most serious pregnancy-related "rash."

♦ Cholestasis occurs when bile (the fluid produced by the gallbladder) backs up into the liver and then into the bloodstream.

♦ The increased levels of bile in the blood cause intense itching, especially on the palms of the hands and the soles of the feet.

♦ Cholestasis occurs more commonly in the third trimester and also with multiple gestations (twins and triplets).

♦ While the itching can be quite intense, there are no long-term complications for mom.

- Cholestasis does, however, have potential implications for baby including a higher risk of preterm labor/delivery, meconium aspiration syndrome (when the baby defecates in the amniotic fluid and subsequently inhales it, causing breathing issues) and even IUFD (intrauterine fetal demise). For these reasons babies of mothers with cholestasis need to be monitored very closely during pregnancy, and early delivery (usually between 36-37 weeks) is often recommended.

Can I treat this?

1). **PUPPS:** PUPPS can't be cured (other than with delivery), but there are lots of options to reduce the associated itching including:

- Oral Benadryl (but beware of drowsiness).
- Topical Benadryl cream.
- Topical Hydrocortisone cream.
- Oatmeal baths.
- Topical Aloe Vera.
- Application of cold compresses to affected areas.
- Oral steroids prescribed by your provider if itching is severe and recalcitrant.

2). **Striae:** These develop because the skin is stretching around your growing uterus (hence the name stretch marks), so they cannot be "treated." Moisturizing, however, does reduce the associated itching, and after delivery, the stretch marks frequently become much lighter and are usually difficult to see.

Old Wives Tale

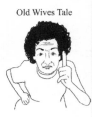

"Just slather on the cocoa butter to avoid stretch marks": Unfortunately moisturizing your belly will not prevent stretch marks, but it can help reduce itching.

3). **Cholestasis:** Treatments for cholestasis involve both mom and baby. For mom, treatments include reducing the itch:

- ♦ Oral or topical Benadryl.
- ♦ Oral or topical steroids.
- ♦ Oral medications like Actigall or Urso that reduce the bile levels in the blood.

Because of the risks to the fetus, closer fetal monitoring should be part of the treatment plan, and that includes:

- ♦ Weekly ultrasounds to assess amniotic fluid levels, fetal growth, and overall fetal wellbeing.
- ♦ NSTs (non-stress tests) that monitor the fetal heart rate over a period of 20-30 minutes.
- ♦ Early delivery (between 36-37 weeks).

TO DO LIST

If you have cholestasis, be sure to check out the "Kick Counts" section of the app and consider doing kick counts at least once daily.

Will this get better?

1). **PUPPS:** PUPPS will get better without treatment after delivery.

2). **Striae (stretch marks):** They do get better. They frequently don't go away completely, but after delivery, they become much lighter and are usually difficult to see.

3). **Cholestasis:** This resolves after delivery with no known long-term consequences for mom. If the baby is monitored closely during pregnancy and delivered early, there are usually no long-term consequences for the baby either.

When should I call my provider? If you experience a new onset rash with fever or intense itching, you should contact your provider.

CHAPTER 4

HOW PREGNANCY AFFECTS THE EYES AND EARS

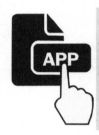

Don't forget to download the Everything Pregnancy app!

1). How could pregnancy possibly affect my eyes?

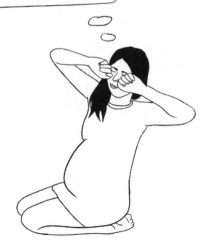

Why is everything so hazy?
Could it be cataracts already?

Vision Changes During Pregnancy:

Is this real, or am I imagining this? No, you are not imagining this. Vision changes during pregnancy are common.

Why is it happening? Let's all say it in unison, pregnancy is a total body experience, and usually, when something new occurs during pregnancy, the hormones are to blame. In this case, rising hormone levels cause increased fluid retention, and some of this fluid makes its way to your eyes and specifically to your corneas. This corneal swelling causes blurry vision.

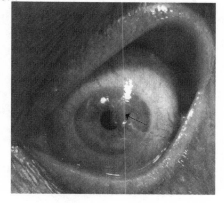

The cornea is the thin membrane that covers your eye.

Tell me more: Like many common changes during pregnancy, these subtle vision changes are usually nothing to worry about. After delivery, as hormone levels return to normal, the fluid retention and corneal swelling will resolve, and your vision will return to normal. Because of these normal vision changes, pregnancy is not the time to get a new prescription for glasses or contact lenses. Many mommies-to-be also find it uncomfortable to wear contact lenses while pregnant because the corneal swelling makes the contact lenses fit a little too snuggly. If this occurs, stop wearing them until you deliver your bundle of joy.

TO DO LIST

A Tip for Daily Living: If at all possible, avoid getting a new glasses or contact lens prescription while pregnant.

Can I treat this? Like most hormonal effects of pregnancy, visual changes cannot be prevented or treated. Luckily, the changes are only a minor inconvenience for the vast majority of women. Just remember, don't run out and get a new prescription for glasses or contact lenses because your prescription will likely change after you deliver.

Will this get better? It most certainly will once the pregnancy ends, and your hormone levels normalize. Fear not, your perfect 20-20 vision will return (assuming you had 20-20 vision, to begin with) ☺.

When should I call my provider? You should contact your medical provider if you experience any of the following:

1. Marked blurry vision or eye discomfort.
2. Spots in the vision or flashes of light.
3. A severe or a persistent headache.
4. Dizziness or severe nausea.

2). Why are my eyes so dry?

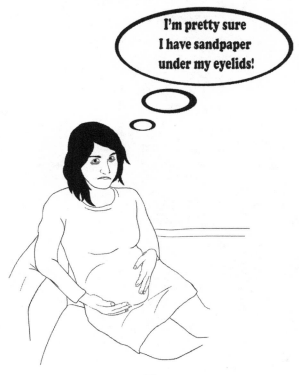

Dry Eye During Pregnancy:

Is this real, or am I imagining this? This is definitely real. Dry organs are a thing during pregnancy, and it's not just limited to your skin and your eyes (oh yeah, there's more! Just keep reading).

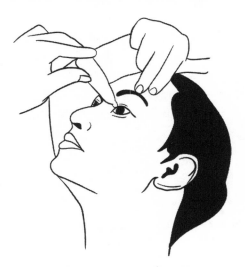

Why is it happening? Just like the hormones of pregnancy cause fluid retention (including in your corneas), they also cause the eyes to produce less lubrication and tears. I know what you are thinking; if you have to retain all of these fluids, why can't you at least make tears? Unfortunately, the pregnant body just doesn't work like that, even with all of that fluid in your calves and corneas, you still can't squeeze a few drops from your eyes!

Tell me more: Your body retains fluid for a reason, and that reason is the health of your developing baby. The more fluid you retain, the more fluid there is in your bloodstream. The more fluid you have in your bloodstream, the more blood there will be going to the baby through your placenta. At least all of this fluid retention serves a useful purpose!

Can I treat this? While you can't force the eyes to produce more tears, you can use eye drops and artificial tears to reduce the discomfort caused by your dry eyes. Just remember, if you wear contact lenses, make sure that you check the label because some eye drops and artificial tears have preservatives that can damage contact lens.

A Tip for Daily Living: Always carry eye drops or artificial tears with you, you never know when you might need them.

Will this get better? Yes, it will get better. Before you know it, your baby will come, your hormones will normalize, and once again, your eyes will produce lubrication and tears.

When should I call my provider? If your dry eye symptoms are severe, and not relieved with eye drops or artificial tears, contact your provider.

3). Are all vision changes during pregnancy normal?

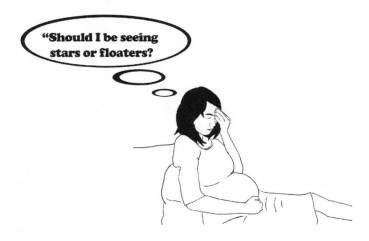

More Serious Pregnancy-Related Vision Concerns: Double Vision, Floaters, Stars, and Vision Loss

Is this real, or am I imagining this? As we have already discussed, visual changes and eye complaints are quite common during pregnancy. They are usually completely benign and almost always resolve after delivery. There are, however, certain visual changes that occur during pregnancy that are a bit more concerning and require immediate medical attention. Normal vision changes during pregnancy are mild (dry eyes, slightly altered or blurry vision), but anything more pronounced can be indicative of a more serious medical concern.

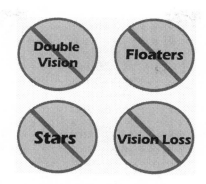

1. **Double vision or seeing floaters/stars:** These can be indicative of more serious problems including pre-eclampsia, a condition characterized by high blood pressure during pregnancy.

2. **Vision loss:** Vision loss is never normal, regardless of whether or not you are pregnant. Vision loss can again be indicative of pre-eclampsia or a non-pregnancy related condition.

3. **Extremely blurry vision:** This is never normal during pregnancy and can also be indicative of pre-eclampsia or elevated blood sugar (diabetes).

Why is it happening? The *why* depends upon the *what*:

1. *Pre-eclampsia/high blood pressure:* Women with elevated blood pressure tend to have more fluid retention. This can lead to extreme corneal swelling, which can lead to extremely blurry vision. High blood pressure can also lead to excessive stimulation of and swelling in the central nervous system (brain), which can cause floaters, stars, or loss of vision.

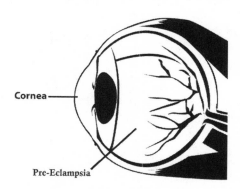

The cornea, which is the membrane over the eye, can become swollen with Pre-Eclampsia.

2. ***Diabetes:*** Gestational (pregnancy-related) and pre-gestational (before pregnancy) diabetes both lead to high blood sugar levels. Over time, these high sugar levels can cause damage to blood vessels throughout the body, including in the eyes.

Can I treat this, and will it get better? All of these conditions can be managed or treated with appropriate medical intervention. For more details, please refer to the sections on Preeclampsia, Eclampsia, and Diabetes in chapters 8 and 23.

When should I call my provider? You should contact your provider immediately if you experience any of the following:

1. Any degree of vision loss.
2. Extreme blurry vision.
3. Seeing floaters, dark spots, or flashes of light.
4. Severe or persistent headaches.
5. Severe or persistent nausea/vomiting.
6. Extreme swelling in the upper or lower extremities.
7. Abdominal pain, contractions, spotting, or bleeding.

4). Let me guess, pregnancy also affects my ears, right?

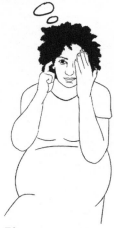

Hearing Changes and Hearing Loss During Pregnancy:

Is this real, or am I imagining this? Hearing loss during pregnancy is not common, but it definitely can occur.

Why is it happening? Well, there are a few possible *whys*. The most common causes of hearing loss during pregnancy are:

1. **Sudden sensorineural hearing loss:** While we don't know precisely what causes sudden sensorineural hearing loss (SSHL), it is presumed to be related to the fact that pregnancy is what is known as a *hypercoagulable state*. That is just a fancy way of saying that the blood clots more easily during pregnancy. It is thought that small blood clots in the vessels of the ear cause this type of hearing loss.

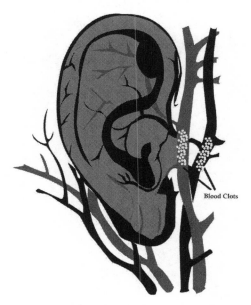

Blood Clots

2. **Otosclerosis:** This is a genetic disorder that affects about 1 in 200 people, and it is more common in women. Unlike sudden sensorineural hearing loss, otosclerosis is a slowly progressive hearing loss.

3. **Pre-eclampsia/high blood pressure:** Some women with pre-eclampsia report hearing a ringing or buzzing sound or in more severe cases actual hearing loss.

Tell me more:

1. **Sudden sensorineural hearing loss:** SSHL occurs over a short time frame, about 72 hours, and it only occurs in one ear. The hearing loss is initially faint, but it progresses over that short timeframe.

2. **Otosclerosis:** This occurs when the bones in the middle ear become immobile, which prevents them from transmitting sound normally. Hearing loss is gradual but can increase during pregnancy. The hearing loss usually involves both ears.

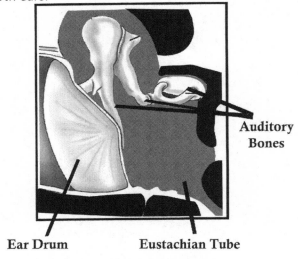

Anatomy of the inner ear.

3. **Pre-eclampsia/high blood pressure:** Hearing changes or loss in women with pre-eclampsia are usually caused by excessive fluid retention or irritation and inflammation of the nerves involved in normal hearing.

Can I treat this? Hearing loss during pregnancy should always be discussed immediately with your healthcare provider. In most cases, treatments are available.

1. **Sudden sensorineural hearing loss:** Because the cause of SSHL is not definitively known, there is no definitive treatment. Some medical professionals will treat SSHL with steroids to reduce

inflammation or with aspirin to reduce the formation of blood clots.

2. **Otosclerosis:** Otosclerosis can be treated either surgically (a procedure called a stapedotomy to improve the mobility of the bone in the middle ear) or with the use of assistive hearing devices.

3. **Pre-eclampsia:** Pre-eclampsia is a serious obstetrical condition that can lead to serious illness and even death. There are treatments for the manifestations of pre-eclampsia (i.e.,medications to reduce blood pressure), but the only cure for pre-eclampsia is delivery of the baby.

Will this get better?

1. **Sudden sensorineural hearing loss:** Some patients report improved hearing with treatment after delivery while others report on-going hearing loss years, if not decades, after birth. The best outcomes are seen in patients managed by an ENT (Ear, Nose, and Throat) specialist.

2. **Otosclerosis:** While this will not improve without treatment, the long-term prognosis with surgery or the use of assistive hearing devices is quite good.

3. **Pre-eclampsia:** Hearing loss associated with pre-eclampsia usually resolves over the 6-12 weeks after delivery.

When should I call my provider? You should contact your provider immediately if you experience:

1. Any changes in hearing acuity or hearing loss.

2. Severe or persistent headaches.

3. Associated visual changes.

4. Abdominal pain, contractions, spotting, or bleeding.

CHAPTER 5

PREGNANCY AND YOUR NOSE

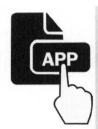

Don't forget to download the Everything Pregnancy app!

1). Why on earth do I keep getting nose bleeds?

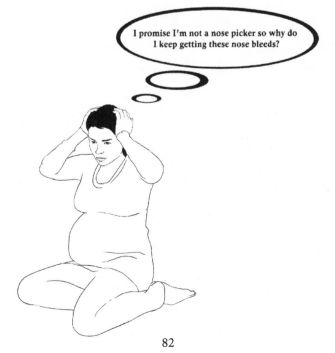

I promise I'm not a nose picker so why do I keep getting these nose bleeds?

Pregnancy and Nosebleeds:

Is this real, or am I imagining this? Okay, let's be honest, some of you probably are nose pickers, but pregnant women still do experience more nosebleeds, so no, you are not imagining this.

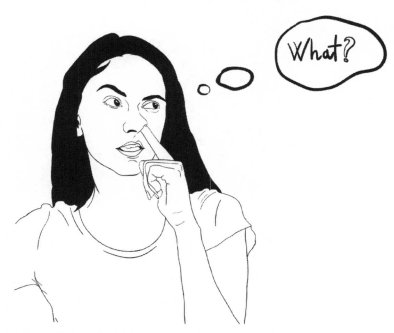

Why is it happening? Part of the beauty of the pregnant body is that it knows precisely what it needs to do to nurture your growing baby. A big part of that is making sure that you have enough blood flowing to your uterus to bring all the necessary nutrients to the baby while also taking away her or his wastes. So, what in the heck does this have to do with your nose you might ask? Well, during pregnancy, your blood volume increases by at least 50%. Combine that with the fact that the pregnancy hormones cause all of your blood vessels to dilate (enlarge), and the fact that blood vessels in your nose are thinner and more delicate than most other blood vessels anyway, and you can probably guess what happens next. These blood vessels break and a nose-bleed results.

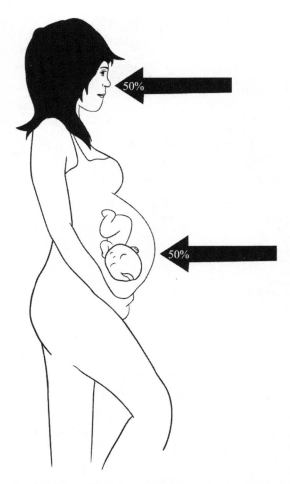

50%

50%

Tell me more: While the normal changes of pregnancy are in large part responsible for nosebleeds, other things can contribute to them including colds and other respiratory infections, seasonal allergies, as well as cold or dry weather. And for all of you nasal archeologists' out there, yes, digging in the nose can also increase nosebleeds.

Can I treat this? While nosebleeds can't be completely avoided, there are things that you can do to reduce their frequency and severity, including:

1. **DON'T.PICK. YOUR. NOSE:** Remember mom's advice, and keep your fingers out of your nose. If you must rearrange things in there, use a moist tissue, and be gentle.

2. **Humidify your environment:** Nosebleeds are made worse by dry air, especially the cold, dry air of wintertime. Consider placing a humidifier in your bedroom and in any room where you spend lots of time.

3. **Keep your nostrils moist:** Keeping your environment well humidified is important, but it only solves part of the problem. Keeping your nostrils moist is the other piece of the puzzle. Use saline nasal spray and topical moisturizers like petroleum jelly to keep the nostrils moist.

4. **Stay hydrated:** This is important for a multitude of reasons during pregnancy, but it also keeps the lining of your nostrils moist, reducing the risk of the blood vessels breaking.

5. **Vitamin C:** Taking 250mg of Vitamin C daily can increase the strength of the blood vessels in your nose. This will reduce the frequency of nosebleeds.

6. **If you get a nosebleed:** Apply pressure for ten minutes to the area directly beneath the bridge of your nose, keep your head above your heart (i.e., don't lie flat), and call your doctor if bleeding persists for more than 20 minutes or is extremely heavy.

Will this get better? Yup, within weeks of delivery the blood vessels in your nostrils will return to their normal size and your blood volume will return to normal as well. Just remember in the meantime, keep your fingers out of your nostrils.

When should I call my provider? Call your medical provider if you experience any of the following:

1. A brisk nosebleed or bleeding that does not stop despite applying pressure for 20 minutes.

2. A headache.

3. Visual changes.

4. Dizziness.

2). Why is my face leaking?

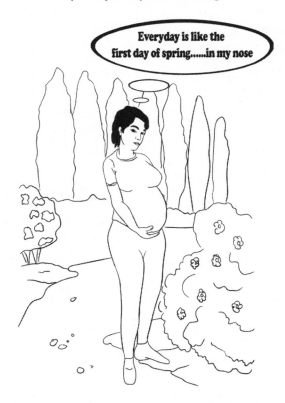

Nasal Congestion, Runny Noses, and Pregnancy:

Is this real, or am I imagining this? Nasal congestion with a runny nose is a very real thing during pregnancy, and as the pregnancy progresses, the symptoms usually worsen.

Why is it happening? Not only do pregnancy hormones cause increased swelling of and blood flow through the vessels in the nose (which causes congestion), they also cause you to produce increased secretions. These lead to both nasal congestion and a runny nose.

Tell me more: While pregnancy often does cause a runny nose and nasal congestion, consider other possible causes, especially if nasal congestion was an issue before pregnancy, including:

1. **Seasonal allergies:** Especially consider this if your symptoms worsen during the spring or when exposed to specific allergens (like pollen or pet dander).

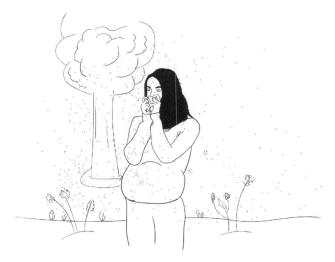

2. **Sinus infection:** If your congestion is associated with a fever and/or facial pain or pressure, it may be a sinus infection.

3. **Nasal polyps:** These are benign tissue growths inside of the nostrils.

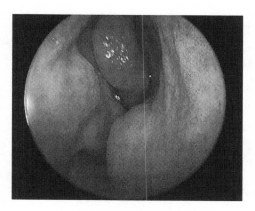

Nasal Polyp

4. **Deviated septum:** This is when the septum that separates the two nostrils deviates to one side.

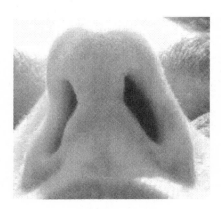

Deviated septum.

Can I treat this? Like most pregnancy-related conditions, there is no way to prevent the runny nose and nasal congestion of pregnancy. However, there are things that you can do to reduce the symptoms, including:

1. **Humidify your external environment**: Place a humidifier in any room where you spend a lot of time.

2. **Humidify your internal environment:** Use nasal saline spray and petroleum jelly to keep the nostrils moist.

3. **Hydrate, hydrate, hydrate:** This is an essential part of keeping your internal environment moist.

4. **Sit in a steamy room:** Steam helps to reduce nasal congestion. If you are one of those rare people who don't have a home sauna, just run a hot shower and close the bathroom door.

5. **Elevate your head during sleep:** Keeping your head elevated with multiple pillows will reduce congestion, and as a bonus, it will also reduce heartburn.

6. **Consider antihistamines:** If all else fails, an antihistamine like Benadryl can be helpful. Speak with your provider first and remember some antihistamines can make you drowsy, so read the labels carefully and only take them when you don't need to be alert.

7. **Consider low dose steroid sprays:** Steroid sprays like Rhinocort reduce swelling and mucus production. Before starting any medication, be sure to speak with your medical provider.

8. **Nasal Strips:** These can do wonders when it comes to a stuffy nose. As a bonus, they can reduce snoring, not that you are likely feeling any sympathy for your significant other's inability to sleep undisturbed right about now.

Will this get better? Like most pregnancy-related issues these too shall pass once your little torturer....err, once your little bundle of joy makes her or his arrival!

When should I call my provider? You should call your medical provider if your runny nose and congestion are associated with other symptoms, including:

1. Fever.

2. Shortness of breath.

3. Dark-colored nasal drainage.

4. Persistent headaches.

5. As always, call your provider before starting any new medication or therapy to get their okay.

3). Why can I smell everything?!

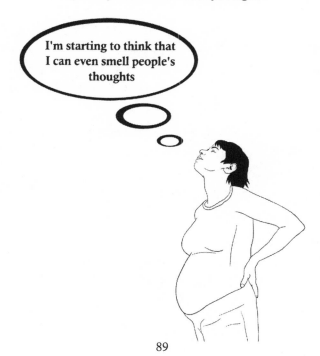

Hyperosmia and Pregnancy:

Is this real, or am I imagining this? Once again, this is real. Almost every pregnant woman has a heightened sense of smell, and while you probably can't smell people's thoughts yet, you probably feel like you can smell just about everything else.

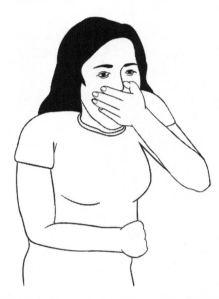

Why is this happening? The safe answer to that question anytime you see it in this book is... the hormones. Studies have shown that pregnancy hormones do increase a mommy-to-be's sense of smell, and the higher the hormone levels (think twin and triplet pregnancies), the more acute the sense of smell.

Tell me more? The technical name for this heightened sense of smell is *hyperosmia*. While the biological reason for hyperosmia is unknown common theories include:

1. Improved avoidance of foods that might be harmful to the baby.

2. Improved ability to avoid breathing in substances that might be harmful.

3. Fostering a closer relationship with your significant other. Many pregnant women report liking the smell of their partner more during pregnancy.

Can I treat this? There is no way to "cure" this hormonally induced condition, but there are things that you can do to make life more tolerable, including:

1. **Keep something that smells of mint with you at all times.** Mint frequently masks other stronger, unpleasant odors, and as a bonus, it can calm the tummy.

2. *Use scentless toiletries* and stop wearing perfume.

3. **Ventilate rooms well**; open windows if the weather permits and put ceiling fans on reverse.

4. **Stay away from foods with strong odors.**

5. **Ask people to avoid using strong scents *in your presence*.**

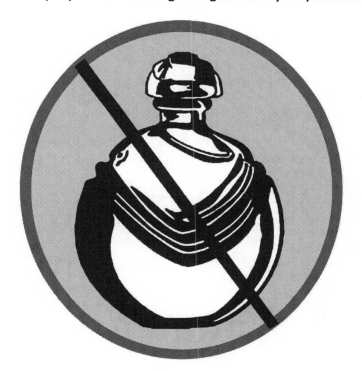

When should I call my provider? If you find that your odor aversion is making your morning sickness worse, especially if you are having problems keeping food and drink down, you should let your provider know.

CHAPTER 6

HOW PREGNANCY AFFECTS
YOUR GI TRACT

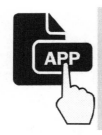

Don't forget to download the Everything Pregnancy app!

1). Why are my salivary glands working overtime?

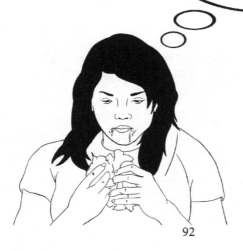

Why am I drooling like a St. Bernard?

Drooling and Excessive Salivation During Pregnancy:

Is this real, or am I imagining this? Excessive salivation during pregnancy is definitely a very real phenomenon. This condition, called ptyalism, is reported by roughly 80% of pregnant women.

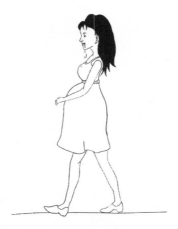

Why is it happening? No one knows for sure why ptyalism happens, but there are a few theories including:

1. Excessive salivation may be designed to buffer the heartburn that most pregnant women experience by diluting stomach acid.

2. Ptyalism may be associated with pregnancy nausea, and specifically a woman's desire not to swallow.

3. The normal hormonal elevations of pregnancy may over-stimulate the salivary glands.

Tell me more: For most women, ptyalism only lasts through the end of the first trimester, though for some it can last throughout the entire pregnancy. Ptyalism must in part be related to hormone levels because women who have higher hormone levels (like those carrying multiple fetuses) also have higher rates of ptyalism.

Can I treat this? While there is no way to completely stop ptyalism, there are things that you can do to reduce its impact on your life, including:

1. **Use a mouthwash with mint:** Mint reduces salivation by drying the mouth. Consider using mint mouthwash throughout the day.

2. **Brush your teeth frequently:** Brushing your teeth, especially with mint toothpaste, will also reduce salivation. There is a small minority of people for whom tooth brushing actually increases salivation, so if this is you, then you will obviously want to reduce tooth brushing to only twice daily.

3. **Eat frequent, smaller meals with minimal starches:** Eating more frequently and avoiding starchy foods will reduce nausea and vomiting, which for many, is tied to increased salivation.

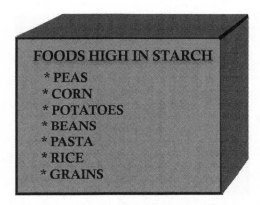

FOODS HIGH IN STARCH
* PEAS
* CORN
* POTATOES
* BEANS
* PASTA
* RICE
* GRAINS

4. **Eat foods high in protein and fiber, and try a few salty snacks:** Foods that are higher in protein and fiber reduce salivation while also improving nausea and vomiting, which also reduces salivation.

5. **Hard candies:** Hard candies, especially mint candies, tend to reduce salivation by drying the mouth.

6. **Prescriptions for GERD/heartburn and nausea/vomiting:** For most people, increased salivation is associated with heartburn as well as nausea and vomiting. Taking medications (and many are safe for use during pregnancy) that reduce either or both of these will also help to reduce salivation.

Will this get better? Ptyalism largely improves as the first trimester comes to an end. For the unlucky few in whom it continues beyond the first trimester, ptyalism will definitely resolve after delivery.

When should I call my provider? While there are no real medical emergencies caused by ptyalism if any of the associated conditions (nausea/vomiting, reflux/heartburn) are interfering with your ability to get through your day or night normally, or if you are unable to keep solids or liquids down for more than 24 hours, call your provider.

2). Nothing is appetizing, and the taste in my mouth is God awful!

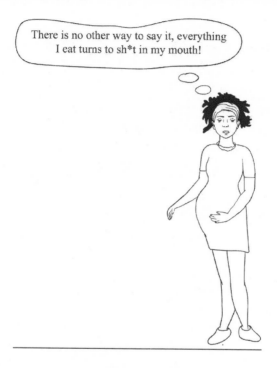

Dysgeusia and Pregnancy:

Is this real, or am I imagining this? This is a very real symptom of pregnancy. Many pregnant women report either having a constant unpleasant (frequently metallic) taste in their mouths while others complain that everything they place in their mouth tastes bad or leaves a horrible aftertaste. This is a condition known as *dysgeusia*.

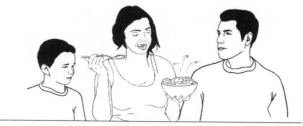

Why is this happening? Like most conditions and discomforts of pregnancy, dysgeusia is related to the changing hormones of pregnancy.

Tell me more: While no one can say for sure why dysgeusia occurs, many believe that it is a protective measure designed to prevent expectant mothers from eating or drinking things that might be harmful to their growing babies.

Can I treat this: While you cannot wholly eradicate dysgeusia, for many people it does improve after the first trimester. Additionally, there are things that you can do to reduce the symptoms, including:

1. **Add sour, salt, spice, and citrus to your diet:** All of these have stronger, longer-lasting flavors that stimulate the taste buds and help mask an otherwise unpleasant taste in the mouth.

2. **Try Ginger:** Ginger also stimulates taste buds while having the benefit of reducing nausea.

3. **Consider changing your prenatal vitamin:** Prenatal vitamins are notorious for causing GI disturbances (nausea, vomiting, heartburn, and constipation), and sometimes something as simple as changing your brand of prenatal vitamin, or changing to a low iron prenatal, can reduce many GI complaints including dysgeusia.

TO DO LIST

Tip for daily living: Go for stronger flavors and try adding a touch of ginger.

Will this get better? Dysgeusia usually gets better after the first trimester, and if not, it will definitely go away soon after the birth of your little bundle of joy.

When should I call my provider? While dysgeusia is not dangerous, some of the behaviors that it can produce (i.e., not eating or drinking sufficiently) can be dangerous. If you feel like your symptoms are so severe that you cannot eat and/or hydrate enough, contact your provider.

3). "Morning" sickness? Please!

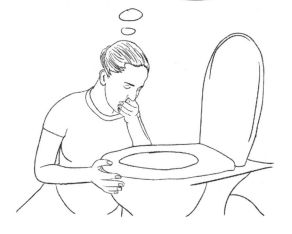

Nausea and Vomiting of Pregnancy.

Is this real, or am I imagining this? I think everybody knows that morning sickness is very real and very common during pregnancy. Approximately 3 out of every 4 pregnant women will experience morning sickness at some time during their pregnancy.

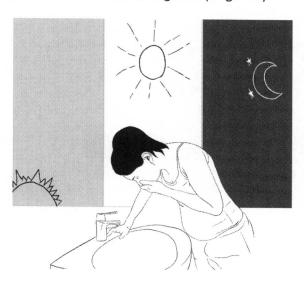

Why is it happening? Morning sickness is one of the first symptoms of pregnancy, and it is likely due to:

1. Normal pregnancy-related hormonal fluctuations. During pregnancy, the levels of many hormones fluctuate, including hCG (the pregnancy hormone that makes a pregnancy test positive), estrogen, and progesterone. All of these hormones stimulate the CTZ (chemoreceptor trigger zone), the part of the brain responsible for causing nausea and vomiting.

2. An increased sense of smell.

3. Low blood sugar.

4. Vitamin B deficiency.

5. Low blood pressure.

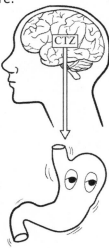

Tell me more? Morning sickness is a misnomer for many mommies-to-be, as it can occur at any time of day, and for many women, it occurs 24-hours a day. Morning sickness is most common in the first trimester, peaking at about 10 weeks of pregnancy, but for a significant minority of women, it persists throughout pregnancy. Morning sickness, which is technically called nausea and vomiting of pregnancy, is more common in twin and triplet pregnancies, and interestingly, about 55% of women who suffer from nausea and vomiting of pregnancy are carrying a female fetus.

Can I treat this? There are many things that sufferers can do to reduce the level of nausea and vomiting during pregnancy. While there generally are few things that will completely eradicate the symptoms, by utilizing some of the measures below, many pregnant women can experience a relatively normal daily existence:

Old Wives Tale

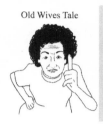

"You just have to deal with nausea and vomiting during pregnancy!": Nausea and vomiting during pregnancy is not just something you have to live with!

1. **Eat smaller meals more frequently:** For many women, nausea and vomiting are worse when they feel hungry or when they feel full. Eat enough to take away the sensation of hunger without producing the feeling of a full stomach. This means eating 5-6 smaller meals throughout the day.

2. **Try blander less spicy foods:** When you have nausea and vomiting of pregnancy, spicy or overly flavorful foods are not your friend. Every person is different, so find what works best for you, but generally blander foods tend to cause less nausea and vomiting.

3. **Avoid deep-fried foods:** During pregnancy, the GI tract is already moving slower than normal, and deep-fried foods only exacerbate this problem.

4. **Avoid citrus, spicy, and/or foods with a tomato-base:** All of these foods worsen heartburn and reflux, which can, in turn, worsen nausea and vomiting of pregnancy.

5. **Try ginger and peppermint:** Ginger and peppermint in most forms (candy, tea, etc.) are common remedies for reducing nausea and vomiting of pregnancy.

6. **Add vitamin B complex:** Supplementing with vitamin B6 and vitamin B12 has been found to reduce nausea and vomiting of pregnancy. Vitamin B6 doses range from 10 to 25mg up to three times daily, and Vitamin B12 doses range from 4 mcg to 25 mcg daily.

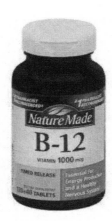

Vitamin B12 supplements.

7. **Consider anti-emetics (anti-nausea medications):** Numerous anti-nausea medications are safe and effective for use during pregnancy. Medications like Reglan, designed for generalized nausea and vomiting, are safe for use during pregnancy. Other medications, like Diclegis, are specifically designed for use during pregnancy.

8. **Chew gum:** Chewing gum, especially gum with a minty flavor, has been found to reduce the severity of pregnancy-associated nausea and vomiting.

9. **Sniff something with a strong (pleasant) odor:** A big part of taste is actually smell, and many pregnant women have a greatly enhanced sense of smell, which can lead to worsening nausea and vomiting. On the flip side, however, sniffing a pleasant odor (especially ginger, mint, or lilac) can reduce the sensation of nausea during pregnancy.

10. **Reduce caffeine:** Caffeine is a stimulant which can worsen nausea in general and especially during pregnancy. You generally want to limit caffeine of any type to no more than 12 ounces per day during pregnancy, and those who suffer from nausea and vomiting during pregnancy may wish to reduce caffeine intake further.

11. **Acupuncture and acupressure:** For many women, acupuncture and acupressure provide relief from pregnancy-induced nausea

and vomiting. Acupressure can be applied three fingerbreadths below the wrist over the large tendons that run in this area. Applying mild to moderate pressure while making circles for 2-3 minutes may help to relieve nausea.

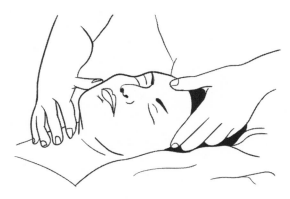

Acupressure

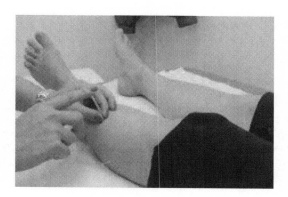

Acupuncture

12. **Start your day slowly:** For many women, nausea and vomiting of pregnancy is exacerbated by motion (much like motion sickness). Setting your alarm clock 5-10 minutes early, and starting your day off slowly can reduce morning sickness.

13. **Avoid exposure to temperature extremes:** Temperature extremes, especially warm, can exacerbate nausea and vomiting of pregnancy. Try to prevent over-heating by taking warm (not hot) showers, dressing in layers, and keeping a fan by your desk and bedside.

14. **Maintain hydration:** Dehydration worsens nausea and vomiting. Preventing nausea is just one of the many reasons that hydration during pregnancy is important. Pregnant women should drink 64-80 ounces of water daily; the more, the better.

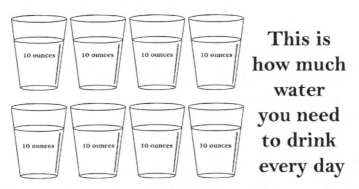

This is how much water you need to drink every day

15. **Lie down, and consider taking a quick nap:** Again, nausea and vomiting of pregnancy is similar to motion sickness, and it can be exacerbated by motion. If you can, lying on your left side while taking deep breaths can reduce nausea and vomiting, and if you can take a quick mid-day nap, that's even better.

16. **Cold food:** Colder foods tend to produce less nausea and vomiting than warmer foods.

17. **Brush your teeth after meals:** Brushing your teeth, especially with mint toothpaste, can reduce nausea and vomiting. A lot of cases of nausea are related to dysgeusia (a persistent bad taste in the mouth), a common condition during pregnancy.

18. **Get some fresh air:** Closing one's eyes, clearing the mind, and taking some deep breaths (especially of fresh air if you can get out) frequently reduces nausea and vomiting of pregnancy.

Will this get better? Nausea and vomiting of pregnancy will definitely get better. For many women, it peaks at about 10 weeks, and by the end of the first trimester, it is a minor concern if an issue at all. For those unlucky souls who have nausea and vomiting beyond the first trimester, it does tend to at least improve after the first trimester, and it will resolve soon after delivery.

When should I call my provider? While nausea and vomiting of pregnancy is very normal, there are times when it can at the very least be disruptive and in the worst-case scenarios, be dangerous. You should contact your provider ASAP if:

1. You are unable to keep solids or liquids down for more than 24 hours.

2. You experience signs of dehydration such as decreased urination, dark or concentrated urine, dry mouth, dry or cracked lips, dry skin, dizziness, fatigue, or loss of consciousness.

3. Your nausea is affecting your ability to function normally (can't work or can't sleep).

4. You lose more than 2 pounds.

5. You are vomiting blood.

6. You have abdominal pain and/or fever.

7. Your nausea is accompanied by persistent headaches.

8. You have a rapid heartbeat.

9. You've experienced bouts of confusion.

10. You have any other complaint that is concerning or out of the ordinary.

4). The thought of food makes me want to puke!

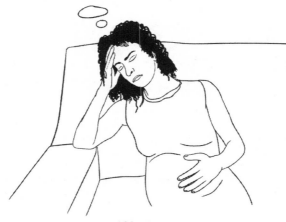

Lack of Appetite During Pregnancy:

Is this real, or am I imagining this? Pregnancy and lack of appetite go together like peas and carrots, and yes, the pun is totally intended.

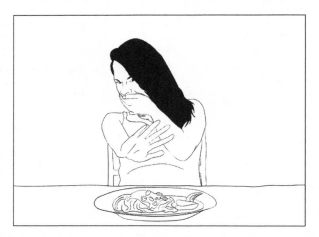

What is this? The technical terms for the appetite loss that occurs during pregnancy (and at other times) are *anorexia or food aversion*.

Why is it happening? Anorexia occurs during pregnancy for a few reasons.

1. The most apparent reason is morning sickness, the nausea, and vomiting of pregnancy, which frequently is not restricted to just the morning. If the thought of food makes you want to vomit, it goes without saying that you just won't have much of an appetite.

2. Hormonal changes are another reason for anorexia during pregnancy (yep, those dang hormones are back again). The hormone progesterone, in particular, causes the muscles of the GI tract to slow down. This means that long after eating, food sits in the stomach and the intestines leading to a prolonged feeling of fullness.

3. The third reason is just mechanical. Your bundle of joy and her or his growing home starts to compress the stomach during the third trimester, reducing its size and capacity. This means that eating smaller amounts will make you feel fuller faster.

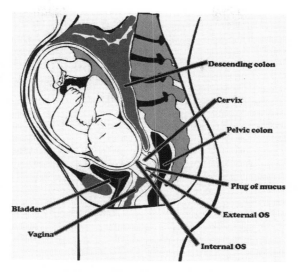

The growing uterus compresses your stomach.

Tell me more: Pregnancy-related anorexia is prevalent with up to 85% of women reporting it.

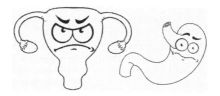

Can I treat this? Because the lack of appetite is due in part to hormones and in part to mechanical compression, there is no way to prevent it completely. There are things that you can do however, to increase your appetite a bit, including:

1. **Eat smaller meals more often.** Eating less food will allow your stomach to more adequately empty itself so that you feel less full after a meal. Because you are eating less with each meal, you will need to eat more frequently. We recommend 5-6 smaller meals per day.

2. **Take the belly belt off after eating.** Belly belts are great for lifting the uterus to reduce pelvic pressure, but in doing so, they actually push the uterus up so that it compresses the stomach more. Consider taking that belt off for an hour or two after eating a meal.

3. **Avoid foods with a strong odor or excessive spiciness. Both of these can increase food aversion.**

4. **Try chilled foods.** Foods that are chilled actually tend to increase the appetite a bit.

Tip for Daily Living: Avoid anything citrusy, tomato-based, or carbonated.

Will this get better? By now you know that like most things pregnancy-related, this too shall pass. Symptoms may worsen as your pregnancy progresses and your baby and uterus get larger, but eventually, that bowling ball in your belly will vacate, taking all of those pesky hormones away with her or him and giving your stomach room to stretch out once again.

When should I call my provider? If you feel that your lack of appetite is so severe that you are unable to eat the recommended number of daily calories, or if you are losing weight, you should let your provider know.

5). Why is my throat on fire?

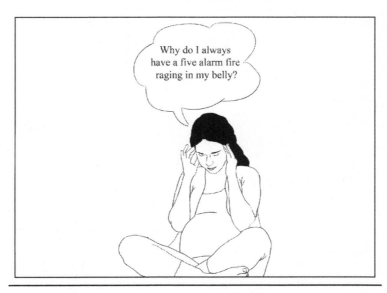

Heartburn and Gastritis During Pregnancy:

Is this real, or am I imagining this? We would ask you to show us the pregnant woman who has never had heartburn, but we won't waste your time because she doesn't exist. So no, you are not imagining this— heartburn is a pregnancy rite of passage.

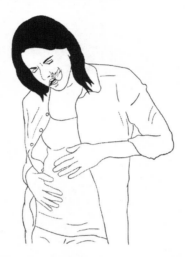

What is this? Many mommies-to-be like to call it hell on earth, but the technical name for heartburn is GERD or gastroesophageal reflux disease. GERD, which is the burning that you feel in your esophagus, is different from gastritis, which is the actual burning sensation in your stomach.

Why is it happening? C'mon, you have to know why by now— it's the hormones! All stomachs make acid; that's how your food is broken down and how your stomach protects you from some of the bad things that you may have eaten. The stomach is designed to contain acid without being damaged, so usually, you don't feel the acid in your stomach. The mouth is connected to the stomach by a long tube called the esophagus, and the stomach and esophagus are separated by a valve that keeps all of the stomach contents, including acid, out of your esophagus. This is where the hormones come in. Those doggone hormones slow digestion by relaxing the muscles of the GI tract. This means that the food mixed with acid stays in the stomach longer and that the valve separating the esophagus from the stomach relaxes, allowing acid to flow into the esophagus. *Voila*, you have heartburn and gastritis!

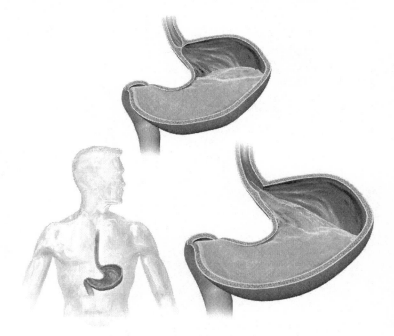

Reflux of gastric contents into the esophagus.

Tell me more: While the hormones play a significant role in the development of GERD and gastritis, your little (but getting bigger) bundle of joy also plays a big role. As the uterus gets larger, it compresses the stomach, putting upward pressure on a stomach that is already full of food, is slowly emptying, and has a relaxed valve between it and the esophagus.

Can I treat this? Luckily there are tons of options when it comes to relieving GERD and gastritis including:

1. **Avoid spicy foods**: C'mon, that one is pretty self-explanatory.

2. **Avoid foods that further slow down the GI tract** like chocolate, fatty foods, and deep-fried foods.

3. **Avoid foods that are acidic** like mint, coffee, citrus, tomatoes, red sauces, and carbonated beverages.

4. **Eat smaller meals more often**; this gives your stomach more time to digest.

5. **Don't eat or drink at least two hours before bed.**

6. **Sleep with a couple of pillows under your head.**

7. **Drink a glass of milk** when heartburn comes. Milk is a base that counteracts the effects of stomach acid.

8. **Try a handful of raw almonds.** Almonds have been shown to reduce heartburn.

9. **Consider adding papaya pills** to your daily regimen. Papaya also reduces heartburn.

10. **Over-the-counter antacids** are safe; just avoid antacids with sodium bicarbonate because this can worsen fluid retention.

11. **Prescription-strength acid-suppressing medications** like H2 blockers (Zantac) and PPIs (Nexium) are also safe to use during pregnancy.

Will this get better? With the measures above, many mommies-to-be will experience an improvement in their GERD and gastritis symptoms. Assuming you didn't have GERD or gastritis before pregnancy, almost all new mommies will notice that their symptoms resolve within 6-12 weeks of delivery.

When should I call my provider? If you experience any of the following, you should reach out to your provider:

1. Symptoms that persist or worsen despite taking the measures listed above.

2. Reflux or gastritis that is associated with persistent vomiting, especially if there is blood in the vomit.

3. Stool that is black in color.

4. Persistent chest pain.

6). Why or why am I so constipated?

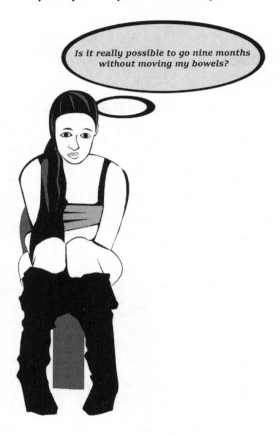

Constipation and Pregnancy:

Is this real, or am I imagining this? Okay, okay, I know that we said gastritis and reflux were a pregnancy rite of passage, but they are not the only rites of passage. You are definitely not imagining constipation; just about every pregnant woman experiences constipation at least once during her pregnancy.

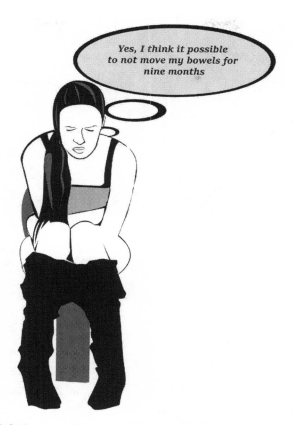

What is this? There isn't a fancy name for it this time. It is just plain old-fashioned constipation.

Why is it happening? Pregnancy-related constipation occurs for a multitude of reasons including:

1. **You guessed it, the hormones.** Remember that lovely hormone progesterone that causes GERD by slowing down the GI tract? Well, it also causes constipation by slowing down the GI tract.

2. **Your growing uterus** presses on more than just your bladder; it also presses on your intestines and colon making it harder (no pun intended) to move your bowels. Of course, as your baby and uterus get larger constipation may worsen.

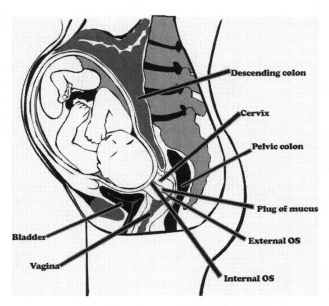

Yep, the uterus also compresses the bowels.

3. **Prenatal vitamins and iron** can also make constipation worse. Prenatal vitamins usually contain iron, and iron is a well-known cause of constipation. If you are anemic and taking supplemental iron that, too, can make the problem worse.

4. **Adequate hydration is crucial** during pregnancy for a multitude of reasons none the least of which is to prevent constipation. Simply put, water hydrates everything, including your GI tract, making your stools softer and greasing the skids, so to speak.

Tell me more: Rarely is constipation during pregnancy dangerous, but it can be incredibly uncomfortable, and it can lead to other unpleasant side effects like hemorrhoids.

Can I treat this? Fear not! There is hope for you and your slow bowels. If constipation is an unwelcome visitor, here are some things that can help move the situation along:

1. **Hydration:** Try to drink at least 80 ounces of water every day.

2. **Get your fiber:** Foods high in fiber like bran, cereal, prunes, and other fruits will do wonders when it comes to softening your stool. The sweet spot is roughly 30 grams of fiber per day.

3. **Fiber supplements:** If you can't get enough fiber in your diet naturally, consider an over-the-counter fiber supplement.

4. **Increase exercise and physical activity:** Activity gets more than just your heart pumping; it also gets your bowels moving.

5. **Reduce your iron intake:** Reducing your iron intake or changing to a low or no iron prenatal vitamin can help. If you are anemic, speak to your healthcare provider before making any medication adjustments.

6. **Stool softeners:** Most over-the-counter stool softeners are entirely safe for pregnancy. Just check with your provider before starting one.

7. **Never take laxatives, stimulants, or mineral oil!** Laxatives and stimulants can stimulate the uterus, causing contractions, while mineral oil reduces the absorption of essential vitamins and minerals.

TO DO LIST

Tips for Daily Living:

• *Hydrate, hydrate, hydrate*

• *Fiber is your friend.*

Will this get better? This too shall pass, and once it passes, your problem is literally solved (get it?). Many women can effectively treat their constipation during pregnancy using the above measures, but if worse comes to worst, once your baby and all of those pesky hormones flee the scene, your bowels will return to normal.

When should I call my provider? You should consider contacting your provider if you experience:

1. No stool for a week or more.

2. Extreme pain with bowel movements.

3. Blood in the stool.

7). Just when I thought it couldn't get any worse, I think I have hemorrhoids!

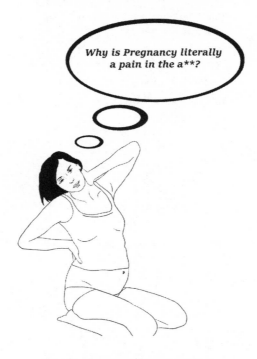

Hemorrhoids and Pregnancy:

Is this real, or am I imagining this? For many mommies-to-be, pregnancy can literally be a pain in the ass, thanks to hemorrhoids. Yes, hemorrhoids are very real, and no, you are not imagining this.

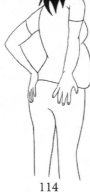

What is this? Hemorrhoids are actually just dilated veins in the anus. Just like veins can become enlarged and engorged in your legs (varicose veins), they can also become enlarged and engorged in the anus resulting in hemorrhoids. Hemorrhoids are just varicose veins in the anus.

Why is it happening? While we blame hormones for everything unpleasant that occurs during pregnancy, hormones aren't the only culprits for the situation going on with your backside. Yes, the progesterone hormone does cause muscles (including those in veins) to relax, which causes them to dilate and enlarge, but your beautiful bundle of joy also has a lot to do with your hemorrhoids. Just imagine putting a watermelon on a straw. That's what your growing uterus is doing to the rectal veins. This pressure, along with the relaxation of the veins, is the perfect recipe for hemorrhoids.

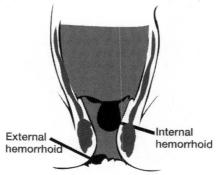

Hemorrhoids can be either internal or external.

Tell me more: Because hemorrhoids are in large part caused by pressure exerted by the growing baby and uterus, as the pregnancy progresses, hemorrhoids tend to become larger and more symptomatic. Common symptoms of hemorrhoids include:

1. Rectal Pain.
2. Rectal Itching, which at times can be intense.
3. Painful Bowel Movements.
4. Bleeding with wiping after bowel movements.
5. Bleeding during a bowel movement.
6. Pain when sitting..

Can I treat this? While hemorrhoids are common and frequently uncomfortable, there are lots of options when it comes to treating them, including:

1. **Adequate hydration,** the more water you drink, the softer your stools will become.

2. **Adding more fiber to your diet** and/or taking fiber supplements will help to soften your stools.

3. **Add a stool softener** to your daily regimen. Double check with your provider, but most non-stimulant stool softeners are safe for use during pregnancy.

4. **Minimize straining** in general (i.e., heavy lifting) and when using the bathroom.

5. **Topical anti-inflammatories** like Preparation-H can actually reduce the size of hemorrhoids.

6. **Use a topical pain reliever** like lidocaine cream to reduce pain. Be sure to discuss this with your provider before use.

7. There is always **surgical intervention** if all else fails. Thankfully surgery is rarely required.

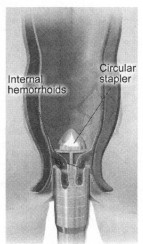

Hemorrhoids inside
Stapler

Hemorrhoids can be banded or stapled.

Tips for Daily Living: Load up on fiber rich foods including lentils, Brussels sprouts, almonds, broccoli, bananas, avocado, oranges and bran.

Will this get better? Yes and no. Once the effect of the pregnancy hormones is a thing of the past and the pressure exerted by your bundle of joy and your large uterus are no more, hemorrhoids will definitely shrink and become less symptomatic. There are some women, however, for whom hemorrhoids remain after delivery. If hemorrhoids do persist after pregnancy despite the interventions listed above, there are quick, outpatient surgical treatment options that work wonders.

When should I call my provider? You should call your provider if:

1. Despite treatment, hemorrhoids are becoming more symptomatic.

2. A hemorrhoid is firm or excruciatingly painful, as this may be a sign of a blood clot in a hemorrhoid, a condition known as a thrombosed hemorrhoid.

3. There are signs that the hemorrhoid might be infected including fever or pus-like discharge.

4. Bleeding from the rectum is worsening or not stopping.

8). Every time I eat, my stomach and back hurt.

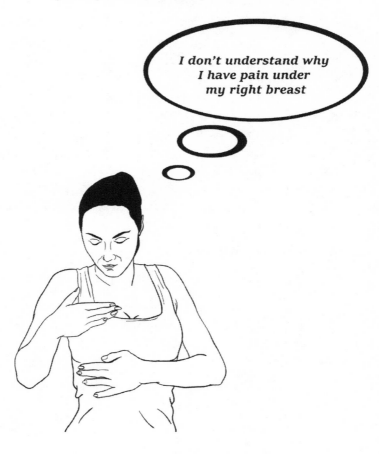

Gallstones During Pregnancy:

Is this real, or am I imagining this? Many of the aches and pains of pregnancy are normal, but there are times during pregnancy when pain is caused by something not directly related to the pregnancy. Symptomatic gallstones are one of those times. While gallstones are not caused by pregnancy, pregnancy definitely increases a woman's likelihood of developing gallstones. So no, you are not imagining this.

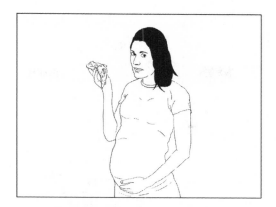

What is this? *Cholelithiasis* is the technical name for gallstones and *cholecystitis* is the name for an inflamed, possibly infected, gallbladder due to gallstones.

Why is it happening? Gallstones are literally little stones that accumulate in the gallbladder. The gallbladder is a little sac-like organ under the liver that produces a liquid called bile. Bile is released from the gallbladder into the intestines when you eat a fatty meal because the bile helps to break fats down. Gallstones form when you have too much cholesterol in your bile, causing it to crystallize. Once you have stones in your gallbladder, they can block the bile from going into the intestines, which causes pain and inflammation in the gallbladder. Additionally, people with cholelithiasis tend to have nausea and vomiting because the fat that they have eaten cannot be broken down properly due to the lack of bile.

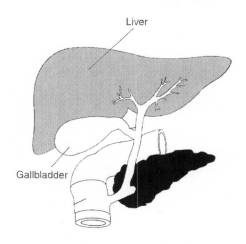

Normal liver and gallbladder.

119

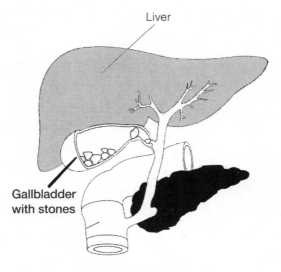

Liver

Gallbladder
with stones

Gallbladder with gallstones

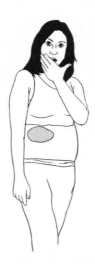

The usual location of gallbladder-related pain.

Tell me more: While pregnancy does not cause gallstones, being pregnant does increase the likelihood that you will form gallstones, and I bet by now, you know why. Of course, it's the hormones. Progesterone slows down muscles throughout the body, including in the gallbladder, making it more difficult for the gallbladder to empty. Other risk factors for the formation of gallstones include:

1. Being female.
2. Obesity.
3. Being 40 or older.
4. Having Hispanic or Native American heritage.

Symptoms of gallstones can include:

1. Pain in the upper right side of the abdomen underneath the breast.
2. Pain in the upper right back or under the right shoulder blade.
3. Pain that develops after eating, especially fatty foods.
4. Nausea and vomiting.
5. Stool that has a a greasy appearance.
6. Fevers or chills if the gallbladder becomes infected.

Can I treat this? While there is generally no way to cure gallstones during pregnancy, there are conservative measures that can be taken to reduce the symptoms of gallstones, including:

1. Eating a **low-fat diet**.
2. Taking **pain medications** as prescribed by your provider.

If symptoms related to gallstones do not improve with conservative treatment, surgical intervention may be required. Surgical intervention is usually performed laparoscopically. This is a minimally invasive procedure that only requires three or four small (approximately 1 centimeter) incisions. Surgery during pregnancy is generally only performed if the gallbladder becomes infected (cholecystitis).

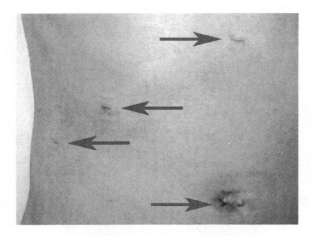

Location of laparoscopy incisions.

Will this get better? Gallstone related symptoms frequently improve with conservative management. Surgery will rarely be performed during pregnancy. Because hormones play a significant role in the formation of gallstones during pregnancy, many new mothers notice that their symptoms greatly improve or disappear with dietary modification and tincture of time. If symptoms don't improve within 12 weeks of delivery despite dietary changes, surgery will likely be the next step, involving removal of the gallbladder, a procedure known as a *cholecystectomy*.

When should I call my provider? You should contact your provider if you experience any of the following:

1. Persistent right upper abdominal pain.

2. Persistent nausea and vomiting with or without right upper abdominal pain.

3. Right upper abdominal pain with fevers.

4. Yellowing of the skin, a condition known as *jaundice*.

CHAPTER 7

PREGNANCY AND YOUR RESPIRATORY SYSTEM

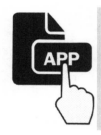

Don't forget to download the Everything Pregnancy app!

1). Why do I always feel so winded?

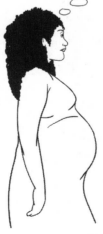

Pregnancy and Shortness of Breath

Is this real, or am I imagining this? Shortness of breath during pregnancy is very real and is almost always normal.

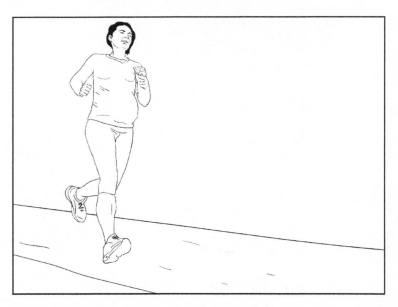

Why is it happening? Shortness of breath during pregnancy occurs for a few reasons.

1. Progesterone: You had to know that hormones were going to rear their heads, right? In this case, it is the hormone progesterone, and it stimulates the "respiratory center" of your brain. This stimulation causes the sensation of "air hunger," the feeling that you need to take a deep breath.

2. The Growing Uterus: Your growing uterus also plays a significant role in shortness of breath, especially during the third trimester when it starts to press on the diaphragm, which is the muscle that separates the abdomen (where your uterus is located) from the thorax (where your lungs are located). This means that your lung volume actually gets smaller as the pregnancy progresses.

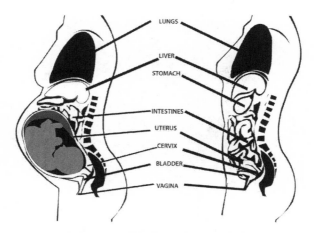

LUNGS
LIVER
STOMACH
INTESTINES
UTERUS
CERVIX
BLADDER
VAGINA

The growing uterus compresses the lungs.

Tell me more: Despite the feeling that your body is turning on you, your body is actually very smart, and it is adapting to its needs and the needs of your growing bundle of joy. Progesterone stimulating the Respiratory Center in your brain causes you to take deeper breaths; this, in turn, increases oxygen levels for you and your baby. This is important throughout the pregnancy but especially during the third trimester when the growing uterus reduces the lung's volume.

Can I treat this? Because the shortness of breath is both hormonal and anatomical, it cannot be cured. There are things that you can do; however, to reduce the sensation.

1. **Proper posture counts:** Keeping your back and chest as straight as possible while also drawing the shoulders back will open your thorax, allowing the lungs to inflate a bit more.

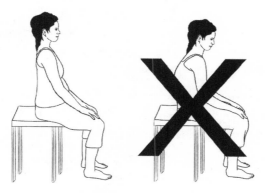

Keep the back and neck straight.

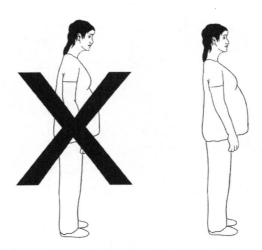

Straightening the back shifts the center of gravity.

2. **Sleep on your left side with your head propped up:** Keeping your head propped up will improve shortness of breath while also reducing nasal congestion and heartburn. The left side is always best because, for most women, their uterus will tilt to the right side. The large vessels in the abdomen like the aorta that are responsible for bringing blood back to the heart also deviate a bit to the right side. Sleeping on the left will keep the growing uterus off of these large vessels, improving circulation and oxygen levels throughout the body and reducing your overall oxygen requirements.

Will this get better? Shortness of breath definitely improves after delivery as the progesterone levels fall, and the uterus returns to its happy home nestled back in your pelvis. Most women will actually experience some relief of shortness of breath during the last 3-4 weeks of pregnancy when the baby "drops" (descends into the pelvis). The dropping baby and uterus give the diaphragm and lungs a bit more space to do what they need to do.

When should I call my provider: While shortness of breath is generally a normal phenomenon of pregnancy, there are instances when it can be abnormal, and you should alert your provider immediately:

1. Asthmatics: If you have asthma and are experiencing more frequent or worsening asthma attacks.

2. Sudden onset shortness of breath: If your shortness of breath occurs rapidly, especially if it is associated with a fever or other respiratory symptoms, this can be indicative of a respiratory infection like pneumonia or other disorders like preeclampsia.

3. The sensation of Drowning: If your shortness of breath is associated with a sensation of drowning, especially when you lie flat, this can be an indication of pulmonary edema (fluid in the lungs) or a rare form of pregnancy-related heart failure.

4. A productive Cough: If you are bringing up phlegm with your cough, especially if it has a deep color or blood in it, this can be indicative of a lung infection or tuberculosis.

5. Chest pain or a rapid heartbeat: Either of these could indicate that your heart is working harder than it should.

2). Am I wheezing and coughing more now that I am pregnant?

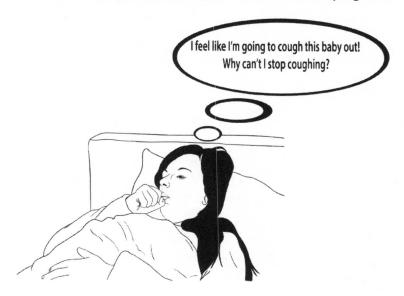

Worsening Asthma and Chronic Cough During Pregnancy:

Is this real, or am I imagining this? Hey, asthma happens! It even happens when you are pregnant, so you definitely are not imagining this. Much like asthma before pregnancy, asthma during pregnancy is different for every person.

What is this? Asthma is a chronic condition that causes spasm and narrowing of the airways in the lungs along with over-production of mucus. All of this leads to wheezing and shortness of breath.

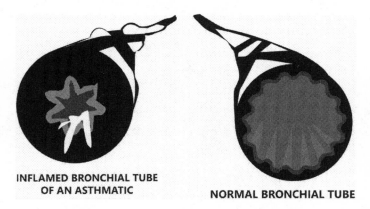

INFLAMED BRONCHIAL TUBE
OF AN ASTHMATIC

NORMAL BRONCHIAL TUBE

Why is it happening? Generally, whatever usually triggers your asthma will also trigger your asthma when you are pregnant. This means that trigger avoidance is critical. For some people, the normal shortness of breath that happens during pregnancy (see above) can also cause asthma symptoms to worsen.

Tell me more: Every pregnant woman's asthma will be different. A general rule of thumb is that 1/3 of women will experience worsening asthma during pregnancy, 1/3 of women will notice no change in their asthma during pregnancy, and 1/3 of women will actually notice that their asthma improves during pregnancy. For women whose asthma improves during pregnancy, you will generally see a gradual improvement as the pregnancy progresses. For women whose asthma worsens during pregnancy, this change is usually most noticed in the third trimester.

Can I treat this? Not only can you treat this, but it is important that you do treat it! Poorly controlled asthma leads to overall lower oxygen levels in your bloodstream, which in turn leads to lower oxygen levels for your baby. This can result in:

1. More severe morning sickness.

2. Smaller babies.

3. Preterm labor and delivery.

4. Pre-eclampsia (a high blood pressure condition specific to pregnancy).

5. Increased risk of fetal death.

So, how can I treat this? Well, first and foremost, you need to devise a detailed treatment plan with your medical provider. Ideally, this is something you would discuss before pregnancy. If that did not occur, this is a discussion that should be had at the first prenatal visit. Cornerstones of asthma treatment during pregnancy include:

1. **Trigger avoidance:** If you know your triggers (cold weather, exercise, environmental allergens, etc.), do your best to avoid or modify them.

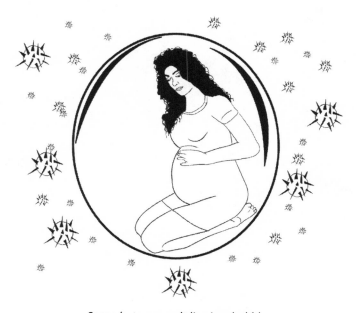

Sorry, but you can't live in a bubble.

2. **Peak flow monitoring:** Every asthmatic should know their optimal peak flow value. This is a measurement of how fast you can blow air out of your lungs, and the more severe an asthma attack, the lower this number will be. Knowing your peak flow when you are well helps your provider determine how severe an asthma attack is and what medications you should take for treatment and prevention.

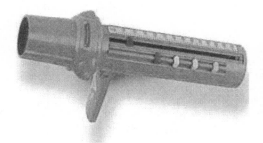

All asthmatics should have a peak flow monitor.

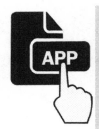

Be sure to check out the Peak Flow Monitoring feature of the app for comprehensive instructions on how to perform your peak flow.

3. **Preventative medications:** There are a multitude of preventative medications that can be taken on a daily basis to reduce the frequency and severity of asthma attacks, and most of these medications are safe for use during pregnancy. They include:

   ◆ Steroid based inhalers.

   ◆ Oral antihistamines.

   ◆ Other oral medications that work to reduce inflammation in the lungs.

As always, speak with your medical provider before starting a new medication.

4. **Treatment medications:** Many medications can be used when you are actively having an asthma attack. These include:

   ◆ Albuterol inhalers.

   ◆ Combination albuterol/steroid nebulizers.

   ◆ Oral steroids.

Much like preventative medications, the majority of these are safe for use during pregnancy but again speak with your medical provider before taking a new medication or changing medications.

5. **Get your flu shot:** We cannot stress enough the importance of this recommendation for all pregnant women, especially asthmatics.

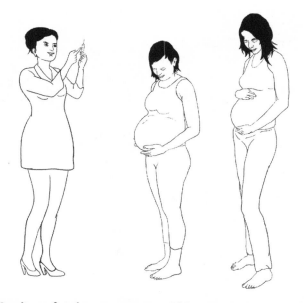

6. **Monitor fetal movement:** This monitoring is known as *kick counts*. There are different ways to do kick counts so your provider may have a different method. We generally recommend that you sit or lie in a quiet area for an hour and monitor your baby's movement. Ten or more movements in an hour is our goal. If you have less than this number, call your provider. If you reach ten movements before an hour, you don't have to monitor any further.

7. **Antenatal testing:** Because of the risks to the baby that we already discussed when asthma is not well controlled, mothers-to-be with moderate or severe asthma should have weekly testing (ultrasound and fetal heart rate monitoring) to make sure that the baby is growing well and thriving.

Tips for Daily Living:

- *Avoid your triggers.*
- *Check your peak flow regularly.*
- *Take all prescribed meds as they are prescribed.*
- *Get your flu shot!*
- *If you have asthma, consider doing kick counts every day.*

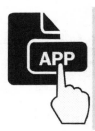

Be sure to check out the Kick Counts section of the app for detailed kick count instructions and a kick count recorder.

Will this get better? For some pregnant women, their asthma improves during pregnancy, for some, it gets worse, and for others, there is no difference at all. While most people do notice an improvement after they deliver, every woman's experience is different, and yours will likely be based on how well you manage your asthma before, during, and after your pregnancy.

When should I call my provider? Call your provider if you experience:

1. Worsening asthma symptoms.
2. Fevers or chills.
3. A cough producing mucus with a deep green or yellow color.
4. Chest pain.
5. Dizziness.

3). Why is my nose always so congested?

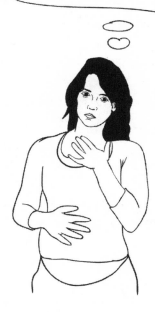

Nasal Congestion During Pregnancy:

Is this real, or am I imagining this? You are not imagining this. Increased nasal congestion during pregnancy is a definite thing!

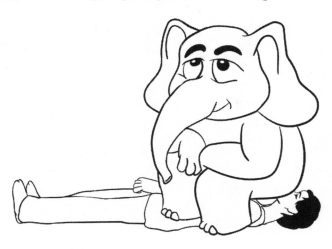

What is this? There are a few reasons why most mommies-to-be experience symptoms like stuffy nose, runny nose, and/or itchy, watery eyes. Sometimes these symptoms are related to environmental allergies, sometimes they can be caused by sinus infection/inflammation, and frequently they are just caused by those blasted pregnancy hormones. And yes, if you are really, really lucky (or an over-achiever), your symptoms may be caused by all three.

Why is it happening? Well by now you have probably figured out that pregnancy wreaks all kind of havoc on your poor body, and no organ goes untouched, not even your face. So why is this all happening?

1. The hormones, the hormones, the hormones: When in doubt, those doggone hormones are always a safe bet. As you move from the first trimester to the second and third trimesters, the levels of the hormones estrogen and progesterone increase. This causes increased blood flow to the nose and sinuses, which, along with increased mucus production, causes some serious nasal congestion.

2. Environmental Allergies: If you suffered from environmental allergies before you were pregnant, you are now playing a game of allergy roulette. 1/3 of allergy sufferers notice an improvement during pregnancy, 1/3 notice no change, and an unfortunate 1/3 notice that they get worse. Whatever triggered your allergies before pregnancy will likely still trigger them during pregnancy.

3. Sinusitis: Sinusitis is inflammation and infection of the sinuses. Much like sinusitis before pregnancy, sinusitis during pregnancy is caused by bacterial, viral, and rarely fungal infections. Pregnant women are more likely than others to get sinusitis because the pregnant immune system is suppressed.

Tell me more: While definitely bothersome, none of these conditions will be dangerous for you, your pregnancy, or your growing bundle of joy. So how can you tell the difference between the three?

1. Pregnancy-related nasal congestion: This tends to be restricted to the nose and throat. The nose feels stuffy, and the stuffiness

at times is associated with post-nasal drip, which leads to an itchy throat and coughing.

2. Environmental Allergies: These tend to be associated with nasal congestion, a runny, itchy nose; watery, itchy eyes, and at times an itchy throat.

3. Sinusitis: Because sinusitis is an infection, symptoms tend to be a bit more severe and include green or yellow nasal discharge, sore throat, headache, fevers, and facial pain or pressure.

Can I treat this? Rest assured, there are things that you can do to get through your nasal woes during pregnancy.

1. **Pregnancy-related nasal congestion:** Because this is caused by those lovely hormones, it is unlikely that you will be completely rid of this congestion and stuffiness until it naturally resolves a few weeks after delivery. There are however, some things you can do while your baby simmers in the oven including:

  ♦ **Use of an over-the-counter saline nasal spray or a neti pot.**

  ♦ Use of a **humidifier,** especially in your bedroom.

  ♦ **Elevating the head with multiple pillows when sleeping.**

  ♦ Oddly enough **exercise,** which by the way has a host of other benefits, often helps reduce or relieve nasal congestion.

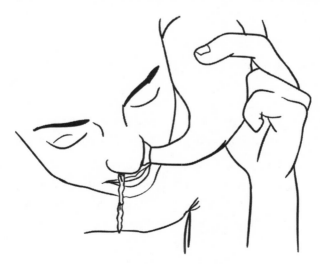

How to use a Neti pot.

2. **Environmental Allergies:** The key to treating environmental allergies is to avoid your trigger allergens as best as you can. Additionally, many over-the-counter anti-histamines and most anti-inflammatory prescription medications do a great job in improving the symptoms of environmental allergies. Note, nasal decongestants that contain pseudoephedrine and phenylephrine are absolute no-no's and should be avoided throughout pregnancy.

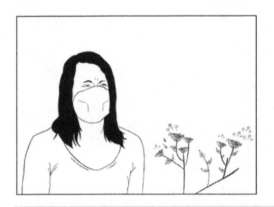

TO DO LIST

Tip for Daily Living: Consider wearing a mask in situations where allergen exposure is likely.

3. **Sinusitis:** Many cases of viral sinusitis will resolve without intervention. In these cases, over-the-counter saline nasal sprays and anti-histamines usually do a great deal to alleviate symptoms. Bacterial sinusitis, however (frequently characterized by fevers) will require prescription antibiotics.

Will this get better? Hormonal nasal congestion most certainly will improve within weeks of delivery. Allergy-related nasal congestion may worsen during pregnancy and improve after delivery. In general, however, the best way to improve allergy-related nasal congestion is to avoid allergens. Sinusitis usually requires prescription treatment and will improve once treated.

When should I call my provider? You should call your provider if you:

1. Notice a sudden onset of symptoms.

2. Your symptoms acutely worsen.

3. You have fevers or chills.

4). I frequently feel more short of breath at night.

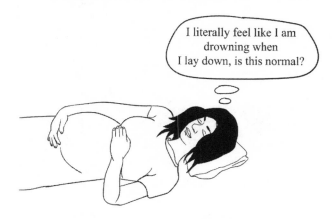

Night Time Shortness of Breath During Pregnancy:

Is this real, or am I imagining this? While this is not a common complaint in pregnant women, some women do experience shortness of breath at night, which can be a potential sign of a serious medical condition. Now we need to draw a very important distinction here. Feeling a little short of breath when you lie down is pretty common during pregnancy. Feeling like your lungs are filling with water and experiencing a drowning sensation, especially when you lie down, is not normal.

What is this? This sensation is known as *paroxysmal nocturnal dyspnea (PND),* and it can be indicative of a serious condition called *peripartum cardiomyopathy.* Women with peripartum cardiomyopathy have an enlarged heart whose muscles pump ineffectively. When the heart pumps ineffectively, it is unable to get adequate blood and oxygen to the rest of the body, including the uterus and growing baby. Peripartum cardiomyopathy is called peripartum because it can occur during pregnancy (usually in the third trimester, but not always) or during the first few months post-partum.

137

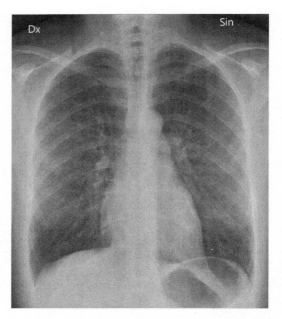

Notice the size difference between this healthy heart and the heart below.

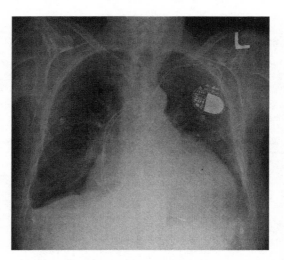

Xray showing an enlarged heart due to cardiomyopathy.

Why is it happening? Peripartum cardiomyopathy is a largely idiopathic condition. Idiopathic is a fancy way of saying that we really don't have a clue why it happens. We presume that it has something to do with the fact that during pregnancy the heart is pumping significantly more blood

(50-80% more) than when not pregnant. Given how rare the condition is (it happens in only 1 in every 4,000 births), there have to be other unknown factors at play. Risk factors for peripartum cardiomyopathy include:

1. Hypertension (high blood pressure) before and during pregnancy.

2. Obesity.

3. African-American ethnic background.

4. Carrying multiple babies.

5. Being over the age of 30.

6. Having heart disease before pregnancy.

7. Having diabetes before pregnancy.

Tell me more: The most common symptoms of peripartum cardiomyopathy include:

1. Extreme shortness of breath and a drowning sensation when lying down.

2. A persistent cough.

3. Palpitations (heart racing).

4. Fatigue.

5. Easily tiring with minimal exertion.

6. Extreme swelling of the legs and ankles.

7. Frequent urination, especially at night.

Old Wives Tale

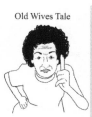

"Of course you can't breathe, you're pregnant!" Excessive shortness of breath is not normal during pregnancy. While shortness of breath is normal during pregnancy, excessive shortness of breath, or a drowning sensation, is not normal.

Peripartum cardiomyopathy is usually easily diagnosed by a few quick and easy tests:

1. **Chest x-ray** to evaluate the heart for enlargement.

2. **Echocardiogram**, which is like an ultrasound for the heart, to assess how well the heart muscles are pumping.

3. **BNP**: BNP or B-type natriuretic peptide is a substance that can be elevated in the blood of patients with cardiomyopathy/heart failure.

Can I treat this? Peripartum cardiomyopathy can be treated, but it is a very serious condition that, unfortunately, cannot be cured. Untreated it can lead to death. This is why early diagnosis and treatment are crucial. Treatment usually involves medications that help the heart muscles pump more effectively, medications that reduce the amount of work the heart muscle have to do, and medications that lower blood pressure. Severe cases of peripartum cardiomyopathy may require heart transplantation.

Will this get better? Diagnosed early and treated appropriately, the symptoms of peripartum cardiomyopathy can get better; however, this condition, unfortunately, has no cure. Patients diagnosed with peripartum cardiomyopathy should refrain from becoming pregnant again.

When should I call my provider? If you experience any of the symptoms of cardiomyopathy during pregnancy or during the postpartum period, you should contact your provider ASAP. Again, these symptoms include:

1. Extreme shortness of breath or a drowning sensation when lying down.

2. A persistent cough.

3. Palpitations (heart racing).

4. Fatigue.

5. Easily tiring with minimal exertion.

6. Extreme swelling of the legs and ankles.

7. Frequent urination, especially at night.

CHAPTER 8

PREGNANCY AND THE CARDIOVASCULAR SYSTEM

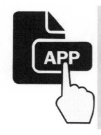 Don't forget to download the Everything Pregnancy app!

1). I literally feel like I have a racehorse running through my chest

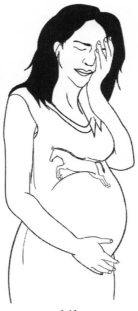

Pregnancy and Heart Palpitations:

Is this real, or am I imagining this? Both a faster heartbeat and the occasional sensation of heart flutters during pregnancy are very real and common occurrences.

What is this? The scientific name for a rapid heartbeat is *tachycardia* (if the heart is beating 100 times per minute or more) while the fluttering sensations are known as *palpitations*.

Why is it happening? As usual, it all comes down to those pesky hormones, but the exact effect of the hormones on the cardiovascular system during pregnancy is actually pretty darn interesting. In case you haven't figured it out by now, growing a baby can be hard work, and your heart is doing a lot of that work. Your growing uterus (and the growing baby inside of your growing uterus) requires a lot of oxygen, and it is the job of your heart to pump all of that oxygen-carrying blood to the uterus and beyond.

Tell me more: During pregnancy, your blood volume will increase by about 50% (up to 80% in pregnancies with multiples), and this means that your heart has to work harder to get that blood delivered to the rest of your body. All of this added effort results in your heart rate increasing by about 25%. Many women notice both the increase in their heart rate as well as the occasional palpitations that come from their heart working overtime.

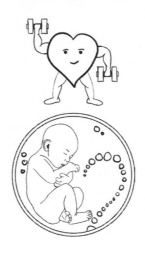

Can I treat this? Unfortunately, this cannot be treated because your body and your growing baby need the extra blood flow and oxygen. There are some things that you can do however, to reduce bothersome symptoms, including:

1. **Meditation:** This can be something more organized like yoga or a meditation class, or something as simple as deep breathing exercises in a quiet location whenever you can sneak away for five minutes.

2. **Lying on your left side:** When you lay on your left side, you increase blood return to your heart and reduce the amount of work the heart has to do to pump blood out.

3. **Reducing caffeine:** I know it hurts (though you should really be reducing caffeine intake to no more than 12 ounces per day anyway), but caffeine is a stimulant that increases the heart rate.

TO DO LIST

Tips for Daily Living:

• *Cut the caffeine to no more than 12 ounces per day.*

• *Whenever you are laying down, tilt to the left side.*

Will this get better? Within weeks of that little bundle of joy deciding she or he wants to evacuate your uterus, the uterus will return to normal size and all of those extra blood and oxygen requirements that pregnancy placed on your heart will go bye-bye. And with that, your palpitations should also go bye-bye.

When should I call my provider? If you ever have a concern or question, don't be afraid to reach out to your medical provider. Now, there are other things that are not pregnancy related that can cause palpitations including an *anxiety disorder, hypertension, and heart disease*, so when it comes to heart-related symptoms, you should always reach out to your provider if you experience:

1. Pain in the chest, left arm, or left side of the neck or jaw.

2. Dizziness or passing out.

3. Severe shortness of breath, especially if it becomes worse when you lay flat.

4. Severe swelling.

5. Severe or persistent headaches.

6. Cough with blood.

2). Is it normal to experience chest pain during pregnancy?

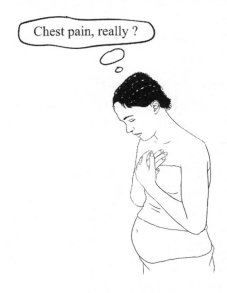

Chest Pain and Pregnancy.

Is this real, or am I imagining this? Chest pain is not a normal symptom of pregnancy, but chest pain related to non-pregnancy issues can still occur during pregnancy.

What is this? There are many reasons why people experience chest pain, including:

1. **Gastric reflux: heartburn.**

2. **Gastritis:** inflammation of the stomach lining.

3. **Ulcers** of the stomach.

4. **Hypertension (high blood pressure) and pre-eclampsia (high blood pressure related to pregnancy).**

5. **A variety of heart and lung conditions.**

Why is it happening? The *why,* of course, depends upon the *what*:

1. **Gastric reflux/heartburn and gastritis:** Without a doubt, these are the most common causes of chest pain during pregnancy. For more information, check out the section on Heartburn in chapter 6.

2. **Hypertension and pre-eclampsia:** These conditions can result in chest pain, amongst other symptoms. For more information, check out the section on Pre-Eclampsia in Chapter 26.

3. **Heart and lung conditions:** While many of these are rare in women of childbearing age, there are heart and lung conditions that can cause chest pain.

Tell me more: The majority of chest pain during pregnancy is entirely benign, but there are times when chest pain can be indicative of a potentially more serious heart or lung condition. Some of these include:

1. **Coronary artery disease:** This is the result of blocked blood vessels to the heart.

2. **Cardiac arrhythmias:** These are abnormal heart rhythms.

3. **Cardiomyopathy:** This is the failure of the heart muscle to pump properly.

4. **Lung infections:** Pneumonia is a common example.

5. **Pulmonary embolism:** These are blood clots in the lungs.

Can I treat this: All of these conditions can be treated, but many are potentially life-threatening, and they all require immediate medical intervention.

Will this get better? This, of course, depends upon the *what*, but with rapid diagnosis and appropriate intervention, all of these conditions can be cured or at least managed.

When should I call my provider? You should call your medical provider immediately if you have concerns or experience any of the following symptoms:

1. Chest pain that does not subside when taking an antacid.

2. Chest pain that comes with or is worsened by exertion or physical activity.

3. Chest pain that radiates to the left arm, neck, or jaw.

4. Chest pain associated with shortness of breath, dizziness, fainting, or extreme swelling.

5. Chest pain associated with abdominal pain.

6. Chest pain associated with a cough.

7. A cough producing green or rust-colored mucus or blood.

3). I know that pregnancy can be stressful, but should my blood pressure be high?

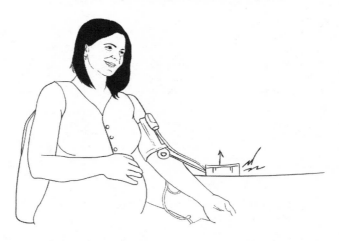

Pregnancy and High Blood Pressure.

Is this real, or am I imagining this? You are not imagining this; Pregnant women can have high blood pressure.

What is this? High blood pressure, also known as hypertension, can occur in women who had high blood pressure before pregnancy, or it can develop as a complication of pregnancy.

Why is it happening? High blood pressure during pregnancy generally occurs in one of three situations:

1. **Chronic hypertension:** This is hypertension that existed before pregnancy. The hallmark of chronic hypertension is that the

high blood pressure had either been diagnosed before your pregnancy or was diagnosed within the first 20 weeks of the pregnancy.

2. **Gestational hypertension and pre-eclampsia:** Both are high blood pressure conditions that occur as a result of the pregnancy and are diagnosed only after the 20th week of pregnancy. For more information about gestational hypertension and pre-eclampsia, check out the section on Pre-Eclampsia and Gestational Hypertension in Chapter 26.

Tell me more: Blood pressure during pregnancy is actually supposed to decrease (see the section on low blood pressure below). Anytime blood pressure increases during pregnancy, it is generally a sign of something abnormal.

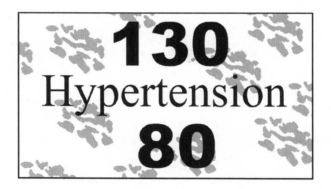

1. **Chronic hypertension:** Most people with chronic hypertension have *essential hypertension,* which is high blood pressure that is not related to any other medical condition. The diagnosis of chronic hypertension is generally made if you consistently have systolic blood pressure (the top number) measurements of 130 or higher or diastolic blood pressure (the bottom number) measurements of 80 or higher.

2. **Gestational Hypertension and Pre-Eclampsia: See the section in Chapter 26.**

Can I treat this? We discuss the treatment of gestational hypertension and pre-eclampsia separately in Chapter 26. Chronic hypertension during pregnancy can, and generally should be treated. The mainstays of treatment during pregnancy are similar to those outside of pregnancy and include:

TO DO LIST

Tips for Daily Living:

1). Check your blood pressure at home.

2). Keep sodium to 1,500mg per day or less.

3). Eat 1-2 bananas every day.

4). Eliminate caffeine or at least keep it to 12 ounces daily or less.

1. **Dietary changes:** *Reducing sodium intake* to no more than 1500 milligrams per day; either *eliminating caffeine* or keeping intake to no more than 12 ounces per day, and *adding a little potassium to your diet* in the form of a banana once or twice a day.

2. **Exercise:** 30 minutes per day of moderate exercise that is safe and approved by your doctor.

3. **Monitor your weight gain:** Weight gain during pregnancy is normal, BUT excessive weight gain can lead to worsening hypertension. Check out the discussion on appropriate weight gain in Chapter 19.

4. **Monitor your blood pressure at home:** Frequently, your provider will have you monitoring your blood pressure regularly at home. We recommend checking three times daily (when you first wake up, mid-day, and before bed) and recording those numbers for your doctor to review at all of your visits.

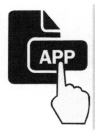

Blood Pressure Log: Be sure to use the app to record your blood pressure at least three times a day. Be sure to share these values with your healthcare provider.

5. **Medications:** Most anti-hypertensive medicines are safe for use during pregnancy, but there are a few classes of medication (ACE-inhibitors, angiotensin receptor blockers aka ARBs, and renin inhibitors) that should be avoided. Your provider will discuss what medications are safe for you to take.

6. **Fetal monitoring:** Most mommies-to-be with hypertension during pregnancy will have some type of fetal monitoring during the third trimester of pregnancy to ensure fetal well-being. This testing could include NSTs (non-stress tests) or BPPs (biophysical profiles). For more details about both of these tests, be sure to check out chapter 2.

7. **Regular fetal kick counts:** We discuss fetal kick counts in greater detail in chapter 2. A kick count is a measure of how many fetal movements you feel over a defined period of time (we usually tell patients to monitor over the course of an hour). Be sure to use the Kick Counts feature in the Everything App.

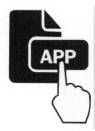

Kick Counts: If you have high blood pressure, your healthcare provider may want you to do kick counts. Be sure to use the Kick Count feature of the app to measure and record your daily kick counts.

Will this get better? With proper lifestyle changes and when necessary medication, chronic hypertension can frequently be controlled and at times, even cured. Sticking to the medication and lifestyle regimen set forth by your provider will help ensure your long-term success. For some, however, chronic hypertension can be a lifelong condition. In this case, following your treatment regimen will do wonders to improve the quality and duration of your life.

When should I call my provider? When it comes to hypertension, you should call your provider if you experience any of the following:

1. Systolic (top number) blood pressure over 140 or diastolic (bottom number) blood pressure over 90 on two consecutive readings at least 30-minutes apart.

2. Persistent or severe headaches.

3. Blurry vision, double vision, spots in the vision, or other vision changes.

4. Severe abdominal pain or pain in the upper right side of the abdomen.

5. Cramping, contractions, vaginal bleeding, or a decrease in your baby's movement.

6. Extreme or sudden onset of swelling.

7. Dizziness, feeling faint, passing out, or seizure activity.

8. Shortness of breath.

4). How much lower is my blood pressure going to go?!

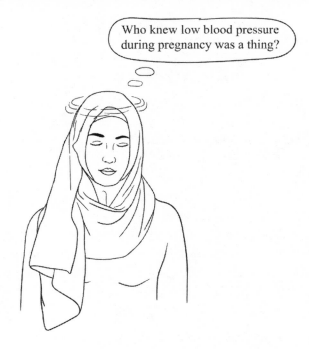

Low Blood Pressure During Pregnancy:

Is this real, or am I imagining this? You are not imagining this. Low blood pressure during pregnancy is an actual thing.

What is this? The scientific name for low blood pressure is *hypotension*. The textbook, normal blood pressure reading is considered less than 120/80, but let's be honest, how many of us are really textbook? Blood pressure varies by person, and low blood pressure is not considered hypotension until you fall below 90/60.

Why is it happening? Hormones, hormones, hormones! Just about every change your body experiences during pregnancy is caused by those darn hormones. In this case, two hormones, in particular, progesterone and relaxin, cause the muscles in your blood vessels to relax, which causes them to dilate and that lowers your blood pressure.

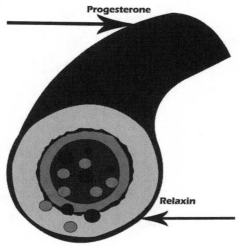

Tell me more: Like most changes during pregnancy, this dilation of the blood vessels actually serves an essential function. It allows higher volumes of blood to flow to your growing, oxygen-hungry uterus and baby. The blood pressure reaches its lowest level at about 24 weeks of pregnancy after which point it slowly climbs back to pre-pregnancy levels. This lowered blood pressure, however, can cause some unpleasant symptoms, including:

1. Frequent headaches: These headaches tend to be mild and usually improve starting at 24 weeks.

2. Bouts of dizziness: Much like the headaches, these tend to improve after 24 weeks of pregnancy.

3. Fatigue: There are many reasons to feel fatigued during pregnancy, especially during the first trimester, and lower blood pressure is often one of them.

4. Passing out: It's not as common, but some mommies-to-be do pass out because of the lowered blood pressure.

5. Worsened nausea: Low blood pressure can make nausea and vomiting of pregnancy worse.

6. Problems with concentration and focus: Many people describe "pregnancy brain," "pregnancy fog," or "placenta brain." Much of this difficulty with concentration and focus is due to the effect of various hormones on the brain, but lowered blood pressure also plays a role.

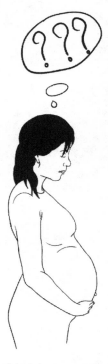

Can I treat this? Low blood pressure during pregnancy can't be prevented, but there are things that you can do to reduce the symptoms, including:

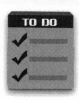

Tips for Daily Living:

1). Stay well-watered: hydrate, hydrate, hydrate!

2). Stay well fed: eat smaller meals more frequently.

3). Keep it cool and loose

1. **Hydrate, hydrate, hydrate.** Oh yeah, and did we mention that you really need to hydrate?! Hydration is critical during pregnancy for several reasons, one of which is the fact that it can buffer some of that natural drop in blood pressure.

2. **Eat smaller, more frequent meals:** The more you fuel your body, the less likely you are to experience the potential symptoms of low blood pressure.

3. **Avoid really hot showers or baths:** Extreme temperatures can make the dizziness that can come with low blood pressure worse.

4. **Avoid rapid position changes:** Quickly changing position from lying or sitting to standing can cause a further drop in blood pressure, exacerbating your symptoms.

5. **Keep a fan at your desk and your bedside:** The dizziness will frequently be accompanied by hot flashes. A nice source of cool air will help both to dissipate more rapidly.

6. **Try to avoid standing for long periods of time.**

7. **Wear looser clothing:** Believe it or not, tighter clothes can make the symptoms of low blood pressure worse by reducing the blood flow back to your brain.

Will this get better? Your blood pressure will generally be at its lowest at about 24 weeks of pregnancy. Beyond this point, it will slowly increase back to its pre-pregnancy baseline. So, in short, yes; with the tincture of time, this too shall pass.

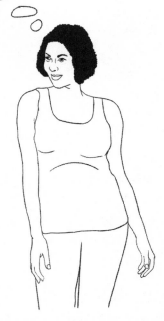

When should I call my provider? You should consider calling your provider if you experience any of the following.

1. Fainting spells or passing out.

2. Severe headaches that do not resolve with hydration, Tylenol, and rest.

3. Persistent dizziness.

CHAPTER 9

SOUTH OF THE BORDER: THE VAGINA/GENITALIA

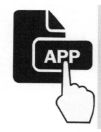

Don't forget to download the Everything Pregnancy app!

1). Is it normal to feel so crampy now that I'm pregnant?

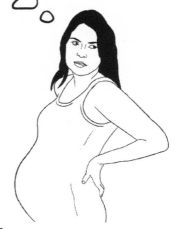

If I didn't know better I would swear my period was going to start

Cramping During Pregnancy:

Is this real, or am I imagining this? Of course, you are not imagining this. Cramping is a very normal part of pregnancy.

What is this? When cramping during pregnancy originates from the uterus, it is known as *uterine colic*.

Why is it happening? Cramping is usually a normal part of pregnancy, and it can occur for a multitude of reasons including the growth and stretching of the uterine muscles, stretching of the ligaments attached to the uterus, or non-obstetrical reasons related to the organs near the uterus, namely the bladder and gastrointestinal tract. The uterus grows from the size of a large walnut before pregnancy to the size of a watermelon by the end of pregnancy, so it stands to reason that some cramping and stretching is entirely normal and to be expected.

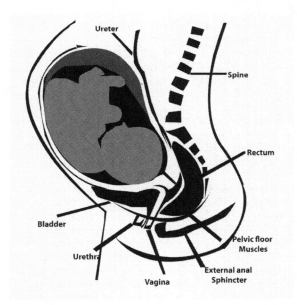

As you can see, the pregnant uterus sits on top of the bladder.

Tell me more: Uterine/ligament cramping generally occurs throughout the pregnancy.

1. **During the first trimester**, you may feel a dull ache or a throbbing sensation similar to the start of your period; this

is often accompanied by bloating. All of these sensations just mean that the uterus is waking up and preparing for the job that lies ahead.

2. **During the second trimester**, you will likely continue to feel occasional cramps and aches as the uterus continues to grow. Additionally, you will start to notice Charlie-horse-like sharper cramping located on either side of the pelvis. This sharper cramping usually only lasts a few seconds, and it is often associated with activities (walking, standing, coughing). This side cramping is due to the stretching of the ligaments that attach the uterus to the bones of the pelvis and is known as *round ligament pain*.

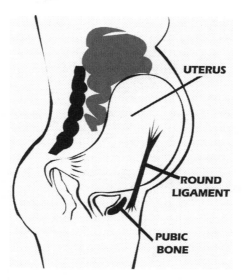

The round ligaments attach to either side of the uterus.

3. **During the third trimester**, you will continue to experience the dull ache of uterine growth along with the sharper cramping of round ligaments stretching. To boot, Mother Nature will throw in some *Braxton-Hicks (practice) contractions*. Check out chapter 21 for more information on Braxton-Hicks contractions.

4. Beyond the obstetrical reasons, pregnant women will frequently experience cramping and discomfort originating in the bladder/urinary tract. Often just having a full bladder

will cause the uterus to cramp, so make sure you empty your bladder regularly. Additionally, our mommies-to-be are also more prone to developing UTIs (urinary tract infections), which can cause cramping of the bladder and the uterus.

5. As if the uterus, ligaments, and bladder were not enough, the GI tract also has to get in on the act. One of the many joys of pregnancy is how it affects your GI tract, and thanks to the hormone progesterone and compression from the growing uterus; bloating, gas, and constipation are all par for the course, and all can cause cramping. Be sure to check out Chapter 6 to learn more about the GI tract and pregnancy.

Can I treat this? Cramping is usually a normal part of pregnancy, and while it cannot entirely be avoided, there are some things that you can do to make it better:

TO DO LIST

Tips for daily living:

#1). Get a belly belt or a belly band.

#2). Empty your bladder every 1-2 hours.

#3). Pay attention to position.

#4). Get a body pillow.

#5). Tylenol if needed.

1. **Empty your bladder:** Your uterus and bladder live in the same neighborhood, and your uterus does not like a full bladder. If you have painful urination or other UTI-like symptoms, let your provider know.

2. **GI cramping/constipation:** See chapter 6 for more details and to learn about the many safe options for treating GI-related cramping.

3. **A nice warm bath:** These are not only relaxing for the muscles and the mind, but you might also find that they help relieve your cramps by reducing some of gravity's effect on your uterus and ligaments.

4. **Belly belt or belly band:** Sometimes all you need during pregnancy is a little support... belly support that is. A belly belt or a belly band is a device that lifts and supports the pregnant belly, relieving some of the stress and strain from the ligaments, uterus, as well as the pelvic and lower back muscles.

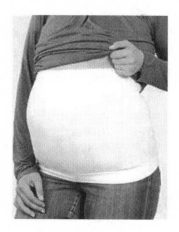

A belly band.

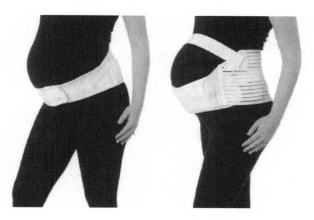

Two types for belly belts.

5. **Body pillow:** Finding a nice sleeping position during pregnancy can be difficult, and tossing and turning can really aggravate those already stretched ligaments. Some women find that a body pillow helps them find a comfortable position and makes position changes less painful when necessary.

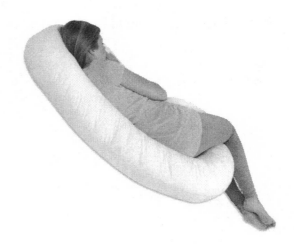

A body pillow.

6. **Position changes:** If a particular position causes more ligament discomfort, simply change positions (we hear ya! That's not always so simple!). Many women find that slightly leaning forward while sitting reduces ligament stretch and pain.

7. **Tylenol:** Tylenol is safe for use during pregnancy, and it can provide some relief from mid-pelvic cramping, lower back pain, ligament pain, and stretching pain. Always remember that NSAIDs like Ibuprofen, Motrin, Advil, etc. are **not** safe for use during pregnancy and should always be avoided.

Will this get better? Cramping from the uterus and ligaments will improve. Unfortunately, this improvement usually doesn't occur until your little cutie pie makes her or his grand entrance (or exit, depending on your point of view). Bladder and GI symptoms related to pregnancy also will improve after delivery though some (like UTIs) need to be addressed during the pregnancy.

When should I call my provider? While cramping during pregnancy is usually normal, there are certain warning signs to watch for, and if they occur, you need to contact your provider ASAP. These include cramping that is:

1. Intense or unrelenting.

2. Associated with other GI symptoms like nausea, vomiting, or diarrhea for more than 24-hours.

3. Associated with painful urination, back pain, or other UTI symptoms.

4. Lasting longer than 30 minutes.

5. Waxing and waning with some regularity and predictability.

6. Contraction-like.

7. Associated with spotting, bleeding, or leakage of a clear fluid from the vagina.

8. Associated with a decrease in fetal movement.

2). Is it time to freak out when I see blood?

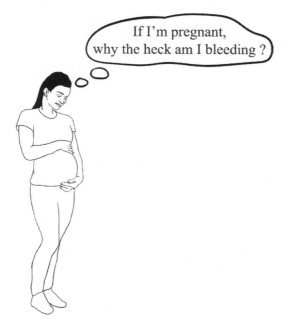

Bleeding During Pregnancy:

Old Wives Tale

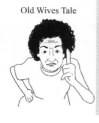

"Everybody has some bleeding during pregnancy": Despite common misconception, there is no amount of bleeding that should be considered normal during pregnancy.

Is this real, or am I imagining this? Vaginal bleeding during pregnancy is not an uncommon occurrence with up to 40% of pregnant women experiencing it at least once during their pregnancy.

What is this? There are many potential reasons for bleeding during pregnancy, so read on to learn more about the most common causes.

Why is it happening? The blood flow to the vagina, cervix, and uterus increases exponentially during pregnancy to support the oxygen needs of your growing bundle of joy. Bleeding during pregnancy can originate from the vagina, from the cervix, or from the uterus.

Tell me more: Let's break bleeding down by the trimester of pregnancy:

1. **Bleeding during the first trimester (the first 13 weeks)** *can be caused by:*

    ♦ *Implantation bleeding:* This is bleeding that occurs when the fertilized egg implants into the vascular lining of the uterus. This is normal and occurs in the first few weeks of pregnancy.

    ♦ *Infection:* Some sexually transmitted infections like gonorrhea and chlamydia, and some non-sexually transmitted infections like a yeast infection or bacterial vaginosis can cause bleeding. Many women do experience more non-STD related infections, especially yeast infections, during pregnancy. Infection-related bleeding usually has no associated cramping and may be accompanied by irregular discharge and vaginal odor.

VAGINITIS

Infection Type	Symptoms
Bacterial Vaginosis	Gray discharge with a fishy odor
Yeast Infection	Thick white discharge with itching and burning, no odor
Possible STD	Copious discharge with odor, vaginal burning

- ♦ **"Miscarriage:** Impending miscarriage can also cause bleeding in the first trimester. Generally, this bleeding will be associated with cramping and will become heavier over the subsequent days or weeks.

- ♦ **Ectopic pregnancy:** This is a pregnancy that is located outside of the uterus, most frequently in the fallopian tubes. This bleeding may or may not be associated with abdominal or pelvic pain. If pain is present, it tends to be on only one side.

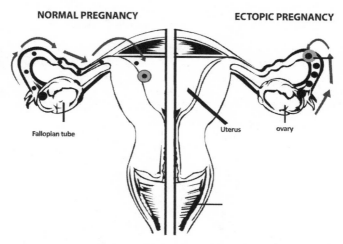

An ectopic pregnancy is a pregnancy located anywhere outside of the uterus.

- ♦ **Subchorionic bleed:** This is bleeding that occurs under the developing placenta in the location where the placenta has attached to the uterine lining. This bleeding may be red or brown and is usually not associated with cramping or pain.

- ♦ **Intercourse/pelvic exam/ultrasound:** Anything that is placed into the vagina, especially if it touches the cervix, can cause bleeding. This bleeding is generally light (with wiping), short-lived (6-12 hours after the inciting event), and painless.

2. **Bleeding during the second trimester (14-28 weeks of pregnancy)** *can be caused by:*

- ♦ **Infection:** Much like the first trimester, during the second-trimester infection is a common cause of painless bleeding (see above).

163

- ♦ **Miscarriage:** Miscarriage is much less likely to occur during the second trimester of pregnancy, but it can still occur up to the 20th week. Much like the first trimester, miscarriage in the second trimester is usually associated with other symptoms, including increased pelvic pressure, clear vaginal discharge, and cramping.

- ♦ **Placental issues:** If the placenta is too low in the uterus, a condition known as *low-lying placenta,* or if it covers the cervix, a condition known as *placenta previa*, painless vaginal bleeding can occur. Another placental cause for bleeding is *placental abruption*, in which the placenta detaches from the uterus too early (it usually separates only after delivery). This condition is associated with bleeding and often severe cramping/contractions.

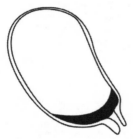
Complete Placenta Previa

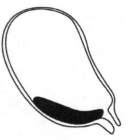
Partial Placenta Previa

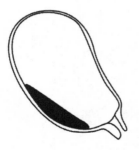
Low lying Placenta

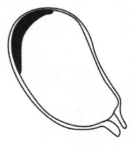
Normal Placenta

Various placental locations within the uterus.

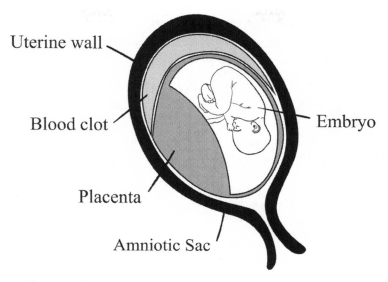

Uterine wall

Blood clot

Embryo

Placenta

Amniotic Sac

Placental abruption occurs when the placenta separates too early.

- ♦ ***Preterm labor:*** Any labor that starts after 20 weeks' gestation but before 37 weeks is considered *preterm labor.* Bleeding due to preterm labor will be associated with uterine contractions.

- ♦ ***Intercourse/pelvic exam/ultrasound:*** Anything that is placed in the vagina, especially if it touches the cervix, can cause bleeding. This bleeding is generally light (with wiping), short-lived (6-12 hours), and painless.

3. **Bleeding during the third trimester (28 weeks until delivery)** can be caused by many of the same issues that can cause bleeding during the second trimester namely infection, placental problems, preterm labor (or term labor), and internal stimulation of the cervix. Miscarriage is not a concern during the third trimester.

Can I treat this? It is important to inform your provider if you experience **ANY** bleeding at **ANY** point during your pregnancy. The ability to treat the bleeding depends upon the cause of the bleeding.

1. **Infections** must be addressed because left untreated; they can cause problems for both mom and baby including preterm labor and delivery.

2. While **miscarriage in the first trimester** generally cannot be prevented once it begins, there are options to make the process easier and safer for you.

3. **Miscarriage in the second trimester** usually cannot be prevented either, but there are instances related to a specific condition called *cervical insufficiency* which if discovered early enough can potentially be prevented with a minor surgical procedure called a *cervical cerclage* (a stitch to close the cervix).

4. **Ectopic pregnancy** is a medical emergency, and it needs to be treated ASAP. If discovered early, it can be treated with an injection called *methotrexate*. Left untreated, however, it can lead to internal bleeding and the need for surgery. In rare cases, it can even lead to death if it is not addressed in a timely manner.

5. **Bleeding caused by the location of the placenta** cannot be treated, but it is important that the condition is closely monitored. If you have an abnormal placental location, your provider will likely give you very explicit instructions to reduce the likelihood of worsened bleeding, including placing nothing in the vagina, no sex, no lifting, and no straining.

6. **Preterm Labor** can frequently be stopped if treated early enough. Even if it can't be stopped, there are medications that can be given to improve the health of your baby before delivery.

7. **Bleeding that is due to stimulation of the cervix** (intercourse, pelvic exam, internal ultrasound, etc.) is not dangerous and usually resolves within hours.

Will this get better? That answer depends upon the cause, but in many cases, the condition can improve with appropriate medical care and intervention (see specific conditions above).

When should I call my provider? You should notify your provider ANY TIME you experience spotting or bleeding during pregnancy. Spotting and bleeding are of greater concern when associated with other symptoms like cramping, pain, contractions, or irregular discharge, but again, all spotting or bleeding should be reported to your provider.

3). How can all of this discharge be normal?

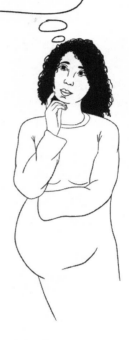

I thought I was going to have a 9 month break from pads, there is no way this amount of discharge can be normal

Vaginal Discharge During Pregnancy:

Is this real, or am I imagining this? Many pregnant women are surprised by the amount of vaginal discharge they experience during pregnancy, so you are not imagining this.

What is this? There are many reasons for increased vaginal discharge during pregnancy, some related to pregnancy others not. *Leukorrhea* is the normal discharge that the pregnant vagina produces. Each woman is different in terms of how much leukorrhea she will produce. Frequently pregnant women will also experience a mucus-like discharge, especially at the end of pregnancy, that comes from the cervical mucus plug. Other causes of vaginal discharge during pregnancy include vaginal or cervical infections (yeast infections, bacterial vaginosis, and STDs). Rarely, increased vaginal discharge can actually be *leakage of amniotic fluid*.

Why is it happening?

1. **Leukorrhea** is the most common cause of increased vaginal discharge during pregnancy, and it actually serves a purpose. Leukorrhea is designed to help balance the vaginal pH (reducing the likelihood of vaginal infections) while simultaneously clearing the vagina of potentially harmful organisms.

2. **Mucus-like discharge** is normal and usually associated with the mucus plug. The hormones of pregnancy cause the production of a thick mucus-plug over the cervix, and this mucus plug regenerates throughout the pregnancy, producing an intermittent mucus-like discharge.

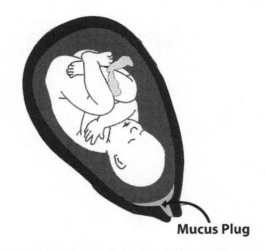

Mucus Plug

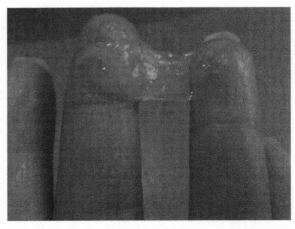

The mucus plug is thick and either clear or greenish-yellow.

3. **Infectious causes of vaginal discharge** during pregnancy include non-STDs like yeast infections and bacterial vaginosis as well as STDs like gonorrhea, chlamydia, and trichomoniasis.

4. **Leakage of amniotic fluid** is a rare cause early in pregnancy, but it can occur any time during the second or third trimester.

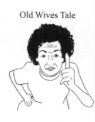

Old Wives Tale

"You can leak some amniotic fluid during pregnancy": "Some" leakage of amniotic fluid is not normal until the very end of pregnancy. If you suspect that you might be leaking amniotic fluid, you should tell your healthcare provider ASAP, regardless of how far along you are!

Tell me more: You can frequently differentiate the cause of the discharge by its characteristics and associated symptoms.

1. **Leukorrhea** is generally a white or pale-yellow discharge that is odorless (or has a very mild odor) and has no other associated symptoms.

2. **Mucus-like discharge from the cervical mucus plug** is generally minimal in amount and intermittent. The mucus will be clear or have a green or yellow color. There are rare instances, however, when excessive amounts of this discharge can be an early indicator of premature thinning and dilation of the cervix, so if the discharge is increasing in quantity, this can be a sign of a potential problem.

3. **Infectious discharge** characteristics depend upon the cause.

    ♦ *Yeast infections* are generally associated with thick white discharge, itching, inflammation, and burning.

    ♦ *Bacterial vaginosis* is associated with a stickier, gray discharge and frequently a fishy odor, especially after sex.

    ♦ STD's are generally associated with a more significant amount of discharge, as well as itching, burning, and odor.

4. **Amniotic fluid** is usually clear, though earlier in pregnancy it can have more of a straw color. If the baby has had a bowel

movement in the uterus (*meconium*), the amniotic fluid can have a greenish color. Amniotic fluid usually doesn't have a strong odor, and it will continue to leak even when you clinch the pelvic muscles that you would clinch to stop yourself from urinating.

Can I treat this? Treatment would, of course, depend upon what is causing your discharge.

1. **Leukorrhea** serves a useful purpose, and you don't want to get rid of it. For some women, however, the amount of leukorrhea can feel excessive, necessitating the use of a pad or liner, and avoidance of darker colored underwear.

2. **Mucus-like discharge:** Is by and large normal and cannot be treated. Again, if excessive, a pad or liner can be used to protect clothing.

3. **Infectious causes** can and absolutely should be treated, for the health of mom and baby. Untreated infections can increase the risk of miscarriage, preterm labor, and cause problems for the baby after birth like blindness.

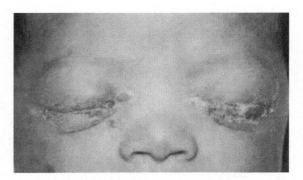

Certain cervical infections can infect the eyes of a newborn.

4. **Leakage of amniotic fluid** cannot be stopped, and later in pregnancy, it is a sign that it may be time for your baby to come. Leakage of amniotic fluid at any point in pregnancy requires immediate medical attention and should not be ignored.

Will this get better? *Leukorrhea and mucus-like discharge* generally will remain throughout the pregnancy. *Infectious causes* should improve after treatment. *Leakage of amniotic fluid* cannot be reversed, unfortunately, but any potential complications can be medically managed if it occurs before term.

When should I call my provider? You should reach out to your provider if:

1. You notice a change in the character of your normal vaginal discharge.

2. You suspect amniotic fluid leakage (clear, straw-colored or green fluid).

3. You experience spotting, bleeding, fever, cramping, or contractions with the discharge

4). You have no idea all of the things that are going on down there!

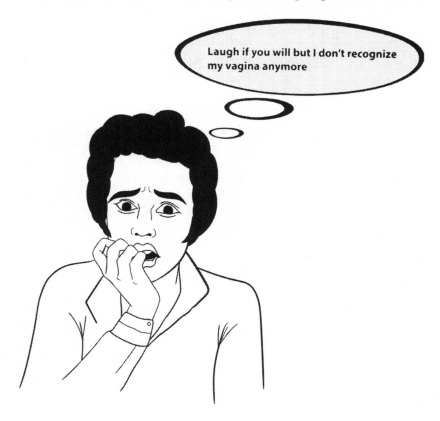

Bumps, Lumps, And Changing Colors Down There During Pregnancy:

Is this real, or am I imagining this? You definitely are not imagining this. The vagina and external genitalia undergo many changes during pregnancy, and lots of these changes can make it hard for you to recognize your own lady parts.

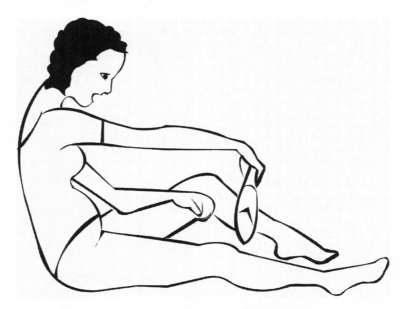

It is a good idea for all women, even when not pregnant, to examine their external genitalia once a month to monitor for changes.

What is this? There is no single "what" that causes changes to your external genitalia, but some common causes include *varicosities* (varicose veins), *Chadwick's sign* (discoloration, usually bluish), *folliculitis*, and *condyloma acuminatum*.

Why is it happening? The why, of course, depends on the what, so here is the run-down.

1. **Varicosities:** Yup, varicose veins are not just for your legs during pregnancy. Pressure from the growing uterus causes varicose veins to appear anywhere below the waist, and that includes that sensitive area right below the waist.

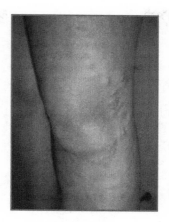

Varicose veins.

2. **Chadwick's sign:** Is a bluish or darker discoloration that occurs on the external genitalia, inside the vagina, and even on the cervix. This discoloration is the result of the increased blood flow that occurs during pregnancy.

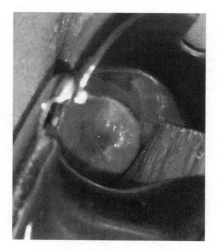

Blue discoloration of the cervix.

3. **Folliculitis, aka ingrown hairs,** is a pesky little problem common during pregnancy that like most other pesky problems during pregnancy results from increased hormones. More hormones mean more sweat and more pubic hair growth. More sweat and hair growth mean more ingrown hairs.

4. **Condyloma acuminatum, aka genital warts,** are more commonly seen during pregnancy in women who have certain strains of the HPV infection.

Tell me more:

1. **Genital varicosities** are experienced by about 10% of pregnant women, and while they are not dangerous, they can cause physical and emotional discomfort.

2. **Folliculitis/Ingrown hairs** frequently do cause discomfort, and if not treated, they can result in an infected hair follicle and an abscess.

Typical appearance of folliculitis.

3. **Condyloma acuminatum (genital warts)** are seen more frequently during pregnancy because the immune system is suppressed in expectant mothers. Pregnancy does not cause genital warts, however, and they are only seen in women previously infected with the strains of HPV that cause genital warts.

Can I treat this? As always, the ability to treat depends upon the cause.

Varicosities cannot be eradicated during pregnancy, but there are several measures that you can take to reduce symptoms:

Tips for daily living: Consider wearing a belly belt or a belly band, especially if you spend a lot of time on your feet, have varicose veins, or if you are experiencing a lot of leg swelling.

1. **Apply ice packs.** These help to reduce inflammation.

2. **Get a belly belt or belly band.** These elevate the uterus, which then relieves some of the downward pressure.

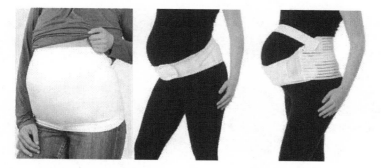

3. **Sit whenever possible.** This will literally and figuratively take a load off.

4. **Lie on your left side.** This will reduce the pressure put by the uterus on the aorta (the big vessel that brings blood back to the heart), which will, in turn, reduce swelling below the waist.

5. **Use good ole Preparation-H.** Hemorrhoids are nothing but varicose rectal veins, and the anti-inflammatory effect of Preparation-H is not limited to veins in your backside.

Folliculitis/Ingrown hairs are not only uncomfortable but left untreated they can become infected.

Tips for daily living: ALWAYS trim and never shave your pubic hair. Shaving creates micro-abrasions that let infection causing bacteria in.

1. **Warm compresses and warm baths:** Both are usually soothing, and both can help to bring the infection to a head, allowing it to drain.

2. **Apply a mild topical steroid like hydrocortisone:** Hydrocortisone is an anti-inflammatory, so it will give some symptom relief while the steroid also changes local hormone levels, making ingrown hairs less frequent.

3. **An ounce of prevention:** Never completely shave your pubic hair. Trimming will significantly reduce the risk of developing an ingrown hair.

4. **See your doctor:** If the ingrown hair does not resolve within 48 hours, or if you have signs of infection (whitehead like a pimple, red appearance or warmth).

Condyloma acuminatum treatment options are more limited during pregnancy than at other times because of the potential risks that medications may pose to the fetus. Treatment options include:

1. **Cryotherapy:** An office procedure to freeze warts off.

2. **Sharp excision:** The lesions can actually be cut off in the office.

Will this get better? All of these conditions tend to improve after delivery.

1. **Varicosities** usually completely regress by 6-12 weeks after delivery.

2. **Chadwick's sign** will usually regress by 6-12 weeks after delivery.

3. **Folliculitis/Ingrown hairs** occur less often after pregnancy, but women who completely remove their pubic hair will likely continue to experience them after delivery.

4. **Condyloma acuminatum** cannot be cured, but there is a broader array of treatment options available after delivery, including topical medications.

When should I call my provider? If you have a concern about any changes below the waist contact your provider. Particular signs to look for include color changes or lesions associated with:

1. Fevers.

2. Redness.

3. Warmth to the touch.

4. Pus-like discharge.

5. Bleeding.

6. Pain.

5). I feel like a teenage boy!

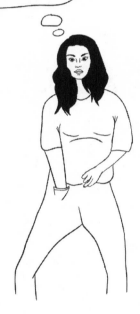

Genital Itching and Burning During Pregnancy:

Is this real, or am I imagining this? Many women report an increase in shall we say... personal itching and some mothers-to-be even report a burning sensation down there during pregnancy, so no you are not imagining this.

What is this? The technical term for excessive itching is *pruritus.*

Why is it happening? There are many reasons why pregnant women experience itching and burning; some causes are related to pregnancy, while others are not. Potential causes include:

1. **Irritation** caused by the normal increase in discharge during pregnancy (*leukorrhea*).

2. **Non-STD vaginal infections** like yeast and bacterial vaginosis.

3. **STD-vaginal/cervical infections** like gonorrhea, chlamydia, trichomoniasis, and herpes.

Tell me more: Generally, the different causes of itching and burning will result in slightly different symptoms.

1. **Irritation caused by the increased vaginal discharge** during pregnancy, or the pads used because of this discharge, generally results in only vulvar/labial (external) itching and burning.

TO DO LIST

Tips for daily living:

1). Wear loose clothes with breathable fabrics.

2). Take wet clothes off ASAP.

3). Stick to unscented detergent, fabric softener, soaps and lotions.

2. **Symptoms caused by yeast infections** are usually either external or internal, and associated with a thick white discharge, while **symptoms caused by bacterial vaginosis** are typically only internal and accompanied by a pasty, gray discharge and a fishy vaginal odor.

3. **Symptoms caused by STDs** (gonorrhea, chlamydia, and trichomoniasis) are usually internal and associated with a malodorous discharge and more burning than itching.

4. **Symptoms caused by herpes**, on the other hand, can have both external and internal itching with burning and are frequently associated with blisters and/or sores.

Can I treat this? As usual, this depends upon the cause, but in most cases, you can treat the cause or at least reduce symptoms.

1. **Irritation caused by the normal increase in discharge** cannot be cured, but certain steps can be taken to reduce the irritation, including:

    ♦ "Use of hypoallergenic pads.

    ♦ Use of a low-potency topical steroid (i.e., 1% hydrocortisone) for no more than three days if approved by your provider.

    ♦ Use of a thicker, barrier-providing cream like Desitin or Gold Bond.

2. **Irritation caused by non-STD infections** like yeast and bacterial vaginosis is easily treated with topical antibiotics that can be safely used during pregnancy.

3. **Irritation caused by STD infections** (gonorrhea, chlamydia, and trichomoniasis) can be treated with oral antibiotics that are safe to use during pregnancy.

4. **Herpes** is a bit of a unique case in that it cannot be cured, but the use of oral medications that are safe during pregnancy can reduce the likelihood of an outbreak before delivery and reduce the possibility of transmitting the infection to your baby during delivery.

And remember, an ounce of prevention is always worth a pound of cure, so be sure to avoid behaviors that can increase the likelihood of vaginal infections, including:

1. Wearing tight clothing.

2. Wearing synthetic clothing.

3. Wearing clothing that is wet or sweaty.

Will this get better? The good news is that the irritation related to normal pregnancy discharge will eventually get better. The bad news is that you will be bleeding for up to six weeks after delivery, so pad induced irritation may last for a few weeks post-partum. Irritation caused by non- STD and STD infections will generally get better soon after treatment begins.

When should I call my provider? Call your provider if your discharge is associated with other symptoms, including:

1. Odor.
2. Itching.
3. Burning.
4. Spotting or bleeding.
5. Cramping or contractions.
6. Sores or blisters

TO DO LIST

Tips for daily living: If you are experiencing genital irritation, consider using hypoallergenic pads.

6). I'm pretty sure my vagina is falling out!

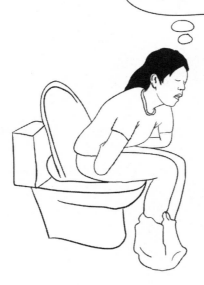

Cystocele During Pregnancy:

Is this real, or am I imagining this? While this is not a common occurrence during pregnancy, some mommies-to-be will notice a bulge at the opening of their vagina.

What is this? This is generally caused by prolapse of the bladder, a condition known as a *cystocele*.

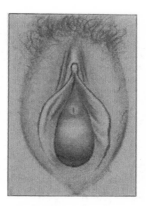

Cystocele visible at the vaginal opening.

Why is it happening? Anytime there is prolapse (protrusion) of a pelvic organ into the vagina; it is caused by weakness in a muscle called the pelvic diaphragm. The pelvic diaphragm is the muscle that helps to keep all of the pelvic organs in their proper places.

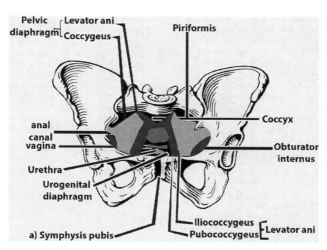

The bones and muscles of the pelvis.

181

Tell me more: Cystoceles are generally seen in women who have had prior pregnancies and are more common in women who have had previous vaginal deliveries, both of which cause weakness in the pelvic diaphragm. Patients with a cystocele frequently report:

1. Increased pelvic or vaginal pressure.

2. Seeing or feeling a bulge in the vagina or at the opening of the vagina.

3. Difficulty starting the stream of urine or emptying the bladder completely.

Can I treat this? There is not a great deal that can be done to treat a cystocele during pregnancy, but there are measures that can be taken to reduce discomfort, including:

1. **Kegel exercises:** These are exercises that strengthen the muscles of the pelvic diaphragm. Over time these can reduce the size of a cystocele. To do a proper Kegel, you want to clinch the same muscles that you would clinch to stop your stream of urine. You clinch for ten seconds and release for ten seconds, doing a total of ten clinch-release sets three times a day.

2. **Pessary:** A pessary is a device that is placed into the vagina to mechanically push the bladder back into its proper location. These are rarely used during pregnancy but are an option for severe cases.

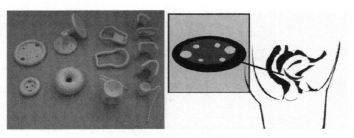

A pessary is placed into the vagina to support the pelvic organs (bladder, bowel, uterus).

After pregnancy, there are multiple options for the management and treatment of a cystocele, including:

1. **Kegel exercises.**

2. **Pessary**.

3. **Pelvic floor physical therapy:** Yup, there actually is physical therapy for the pelvic floor muscles, and for some women with milder cystoceles, this is a viable non-surgical option.

4. **Surgical intervention:** Generally, an outpatient procedure that requires only internal or very small external incisions to lift the bladder back to its normal anatomical position.

Will this get better? Generally, cystoceles do not improve over time unless treated. As a matter of fact, with subsequent pregnancies and deliveries, combined with the effect of perimenopausal and postmenopausal hormonal fluctuations, cystoceles may actually worsen over time.

When should I call my provider? You should call your provider if:

1. The bulge is causing significant pain or discomfort.

2. You are having trouble urinating normally.

3. You have UTI (Urinary Tract Infection) symptoms.

4. There is bleeding present.

7). Is my vagina more open now?

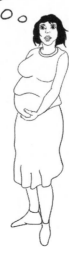

It is possible that my vagina is more open now that I am pregnant?

Vaginal Relaxation During Pregnancy:

Is this real, or am I imagining this? While this is something that many moms- to-be rarely discuss, it can happen, and you are not imagining this.

What is this? Pelvic floor relaxation is a relaxation of the muscles that support the pelvic organs (uterus, bowel, and bladder).

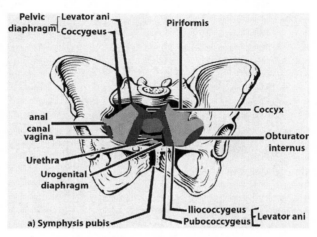

The muscles of the pelvic diaphragm support the pelvic organs, including the uterus, bladder, and bowels.

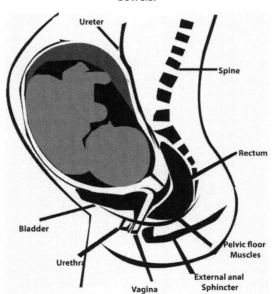

During pregnancy, the growing uterus puts pressure on the pelvic diaphragm.

Why is it happening? The human body is an amazingly adaptable specimen, and the pregnant human body makes some pretty big adaptations to allow your little bundle of joy to grow and eventually escape the confines of your comfy womb. As you can imagine, squeezing a 7 ½ pound human being through your pelvis and out of your vagina requires some physical changes on the part of your pelvis and genital tract.

Tell me more: The pregnancy hormone progesterone causes relaxation of smooth muscle; these are the muscles that you cannot control. The smooth muscles in the pelvis and lining the vagina relax in response to surging progesterone levels, which causes relaxation of the vagina and the vaginal opening. Add to that the pressure exerted by twelve pounds of baby, amniotic fluid, and uterus and the relaxing effect on the pelvis and vagina is even greater.

Can I treat this? This is a normal part of pregnancy, but some things can be done to lessen the effect, including:

1. **Wear a belly belt or belly band:** This lifts the uterus and reduces pelvic pressure from the growing uterus.

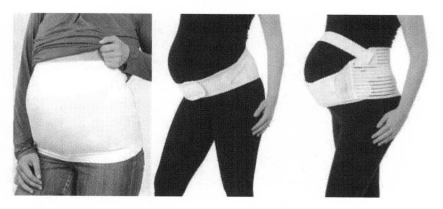

2. **Take a load off:** While most pregnant women should remain active (it's better for you and baby), taking a load off every now and again goes a long way towards reducing the pressure that can cause vaginal relaxation.

Will this get better? This too shall pass, for the most part. After your body's big finish, your hormone levels will start to normalize. Combine these normalizing hormones with the decrease in pelvic pressure that comes with your uterus returning to its normal size and the vaginal relaxation should mostly resolve within 6-12 weeks of delivery. Some women do report that their vagina after birth is not the same as it was before delivery, but for many, the changes are mild.

When should I call my provider? You should call your provider if the pressure:

1. Is acutely worse.

2. Is associated with spotting, bleeding, or leakage of clear fluid from the vagina.

3. Is accompanied by pelvic pain, cramping, or contractions.

CHAPTER 10

PREGNANCY AND YOUR BREASTS

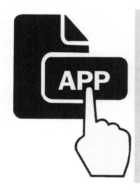

Don't forget to download the Everything Pregnancy app!

1). Why does it feel like my breasts are on fire?

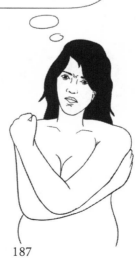

Touch my breasts and I'll kill you

Breast Pain and Enlargement During Pregnancy:

Is this real, or am I imagining this? These are very real and very common complaints of pregnancy, so no, you are not imagining this.

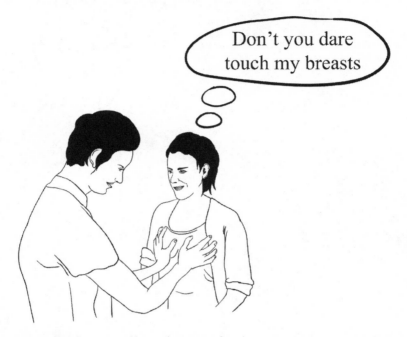

What is this? The technical name for breast pain is *mastalgia* or *mastodynia*.

Why is it happening? Surely, we don't have to say it by now, but just for the sake of completeness we're going to say it anyway, it's the hormones, silly! Your body is a melting pot of hormones that affect your breasts including:

1. Estrogen.
2. Progesterone.
3. hCG.
4. Relaxin.
5. Prolactin.

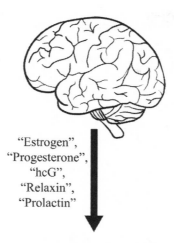

"Estrogen",
"Progesterone",
"hcG",
"Relaxin",
"Prolactin"

Estrogen, progesterone, and prolactin are preparing your breasts for *lactation* (milk production) by stimulating breast growth, increasing blood flow to your breasts, and causing a proliferation of the glands that will be necessary for lactation. While miraculous and necessary, this hard work can be painful.

Tell me more: While every mommy-to-be's pregnancy is different, for the majority of women breast pain is at its most severe during the first trimester (first 14 weeks of pregnancy), usually improving during the second trimester, and returning, but to a lesser extent, during the third trimester (after 28 weeks). Breast growth, on the other hand, tends to occur gradually throughout the pregnancy.

Can I treat this? You can't completely get rid of breast pain, but there are lots of things that you can do to significantly reduce the pain, allowing you to get through your day and night more comfortably. So, what can you do?

TO DO LIST

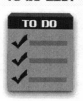

Tips for Daily Living:

#1. Don't touch or stimulate your breasts.

#2. Keep your breasts well supported.

#3. Ice the ladies if needed.

#4. Stick to breathable fibers.

#5. If all else fails, ditch the bra!

189

1. **Wear a well-fitted bra or sports bra**. Likely all of your bras will be tighter given the increased size of your breasts, but buying a few well-fitted bras will do wonders. And for the love of God, avoid underwire! Underwire will only make the situation worse!

2. **Maternity bras** are actually a thing. If a well-fitted bra doesn't help, consider buying a maternity bra.

3. **Cotton, Cotton, Cotton,** Synthetic materials are not your friend during pregnancy, and they will only make breast discomfort worse.

4. **If all else fails, consider going bra-less**. For the majority of women, a well-fitted bra does the trick, but for some women, the breasts are so exquisitely tender that anything touching them causes pain. In this case, going bra-less may do the trick.

5. **Ice packs:** It may seem a bit strange but placing an ice pack in that well-fitted bra provides many expectant mothers with a great deal of relief.

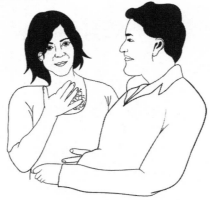

6. **Tylenol.** If all else fails, and the pain is not otherwise relieved, a little Tylenol from time to time is okay.

Will this get better?

1. **Pregnancy-related breast pain** will always get better; it's just a matter of when. Most women notice lots of relief during the second trimester of pregnancy, though some breast pain

190

will likely return during the third trimester. Now we won't lie to you, many nursing mothers will experience breast pain at some point during their nursing career, but much like breast pain during pregnancy, there are tons of things that can help, and we all know that the benefits of nursing for both mom and baby are definitely worth it in the end.

2. **Breast enlargement** will subside within 6-12 weeks of delivery for women who choose not to breastfeed. For new mothers who do breastfeed, and we highly encourage breastfeeding as it is best for mom and baby, breast enlargement usually remains for the duration of breastfeeding.

When should I call my provider? While you should contact your provider anytime you have a question or concern, you should definitely reach out to your provider if you experience any of the following:

1. Sudden onset of breast pain.

2. Pain or enlargement associated with redness or a palpable lump or mass.

3. Fever.

4. Bloody nipple discharge.

2). Why are my breasts leaking long before there is a baby to feed?

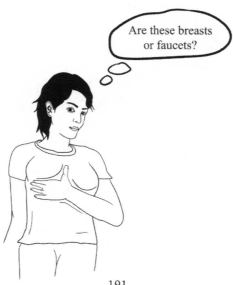

Breast Leakage During Pregnancy:

Is this real, or am I imagining this? You are not imagining this; leakage from the nipples is a very real and very common complaint during pregnancy.

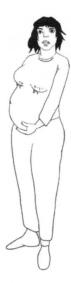

Why is it happening? We are mammals after all, and the mam in mammal stands for mammary. Translation, your breasts are designed to serve a very important purpose: the production of nourishing, life-sustaining milk for your baby.

Old Wives Tale

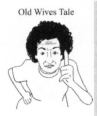

"If you don't leak you won't be able to breastfeed": *If your breasts don't leak during pregnancy, you will be unable to breastfeed. Not true! Even if you don't notice nipple leakage during pregnancy, you most certainly can still breastfeed.*

Old Wives Tale

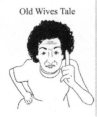

"Leaking means you are going to deliver early": If you experience breast leakage early in pregnancy, you will deliver early. Another Old Wives' Tale, starting lactation earlier during pregnancy does NOT mean that you will deliver early.

Tell me more: Most nipple discharge during pregnancy is related to lactation, the process by which the breasts produce milk. While almost every woman will experience some leakage from her nipples at some point during pregnancy, when (or even if) this will occur is different from mommy to mommy. Generally, you will notice a thicker, clear fluid known as *colostrum*. Colostrum is the protein-rich precursor to breast milk that is easier for your baby to digest. Colostrum production can start as early as 14 weeks of pregnancy (end of the first trimester) though you may not notice it at all. Some women, especially those who have breastfed in the past, may notice actual milk production before delivery, but many will not. If you do not experience nipple leakage or discharge during pregnancy, fear not! Production of colostrum or milk, or the lack thereof, during pregnancy is by no means an indication of your ability to successfully breastfeed your bundle of joy.

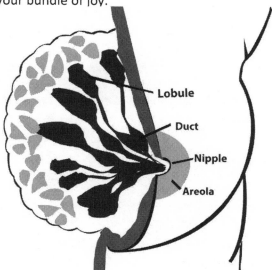

Lobule

Duct

Nipple

Areola

Anatomy of the breast: Milk is produced in the
lobules and passes through the ducts.

Can I treat this? There is no need to treat breast leakage during pregnancy because it's normal. Having said that, experiencing breasts that leak whenever and wherever they want can be annoying, especially because they seem to have radar for your favorite pieces of clothing.

Here are some things that you can try to lessen the burden caused by your leaky breasts:

1. **Wear nursing pads.** These pads cover the nipples and trust us; they will be your breast friends when you are nursing. The good news is that you don't have to wait until you deliver to use them, and they do wonders when it comes to protecting your clothing.

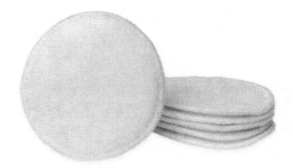

Nursing Pads.

2. **Hands off the goods!** Stimulating the breasts will stimulate further production of colostrum or milk, so minimize stimulation. We are talking about any form of, by the way, not just touching the breasts. Many women, in fact, choose to shower with their back to the water to prevent breast stimulation while they bathe.

TO DO LIST

Tip for Daily Living: Consider investing in nursing pads earlier rather than later.

Will this get better? Your mom isn't still lactating, so this will definitely get better. During pregnancy, however, the discharge will likely increase as you get closer to the time of delivery. After delivery, lactation will continue as long as you choose to breastfeed your baby and even for a few weeks after you wean her or him. If you decide not to breastfeed, the discharge should improve within 6-12 weeks of delivery.

When should I call my provider? You should call your provider if:

1. The discharge has a color other than white, pale yellow, or pale green.
2. You see blood in the discharge.
3. You experience fevers, redness, breast warmth, or a lump or bump in the breast.

Old Wives Tale

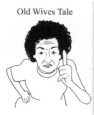

*"**Big breasts mean more milk**": Larger breasts mean more milk production. This is another Old Wives' Tale; larger breasts do not mean more milk production.*

3). I'm pretty sure my breasts and nipples are changing colors!

Will my breasts really become every color of the rainbow?

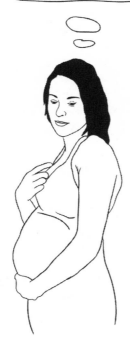

Breast Color Changes During Pregnancy:

Is this real, or am I imagining this? Color changes of the breasts, nipples, and areolas during pregnancy are a very real phenomenon, so you are not imagining this.

What is this? There is no technical name for the color changes that women experience during pregnancy, so give it whatever nickname you like!

Why is it happening? Your good old friend, hormones cause breast and nipple/areola color changes during pregnancy.

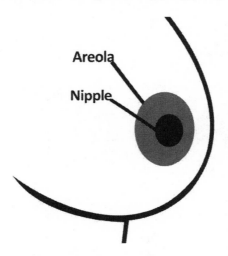

Tell me more: While hormones are responsible for many of your pregnancy discomforts, the hormones of pregnancy really do serve an important purpose when it comes to your breasts, preparing them for lactation. A big part of this preparation involves increasing blood flow to your breasts. So, how exactly do these hormonal changes relate to some of the color changes you are seeing?

1. **Darker or pinker breasts:** The increased blood flow causes the breasts of darker skinned women to become darker while the breasts of fairer skinned women become pinker.

2. **Blue discoloration/prominent veins:** The enlarging veins necessary to support the increased blood flow frequently cause a bluish discoloration.

3. **Darker areola:** The hCG hormone that is produced during pregnancy is very similar to a hormone called MSH that is responsible for generalized pigmentation. This is why many pregnant women notice facial discoloration known as *melasma* (the so-called mask of pregnancy), a darkening of the *linea alba* (the dark line running down the belly), and this is also why many pregnant women notice that their areolas darken and enlarge.

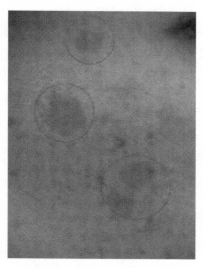

Melasma (mask of pregnancy).

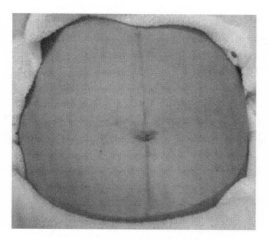

Linea nigra of pregnancy.

Can I treat this? Sorry, most breast changes, including color changes, are just part of the territory. Excessive sun exposure can, however, exacerbate these skin color changes, so consider keeping the ladies undercover.

Will this get better?

1. **The darker discoloration of the face, abdomen and nipples/ areola** caused by hCG levels may slightly improve during the third trimester as hCG levels naturally decrease. If it doesn't, don't fret; for some women, this improvement just doesn't occur.

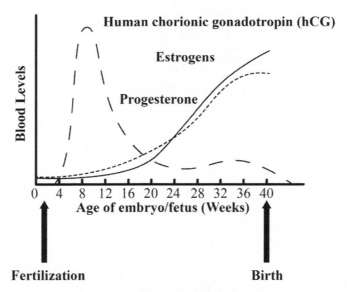

Typical hormonal trends during pregnancy.

2. **Other color changes related to increased blood flow** (darker or pinker breasts) and prominent veins (bluish discoloration) usually do not improve during pregnancy. If you choose not to breastfeed, these changes will be gone by 6-12 weeks after delivery. If you decide to breastfeed, the changes will likely hang around until you wean your bundle of joy.

When should I call my provider? You should call your provider if your breasts are:

1. Red or inflamed.
2. If you feel a lump or a bump.

4). Why do my breasts feel so lumpy?

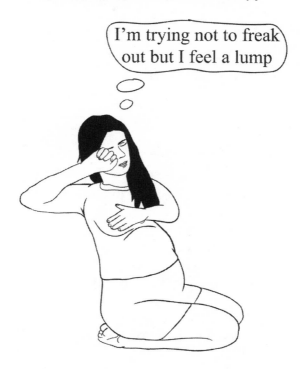

Breast Lumps During Pregnancy:

Is this real, or am I imagining this? While breast lumps during pregnancy can certainly be normal, they should always be examined by your provider.

What is this? There are many causes of breast lumps during pregnancy, and most are related to the pregnancy or lactation, including:

1. **Enlargement of the breast glands.**
2. **A blocked milk duct.**
3. **A breast infection** including *mastitis* or an abscess.

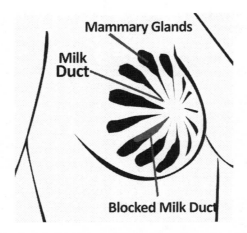

A palpable cord in the breast usually characterizes a blocked duct.

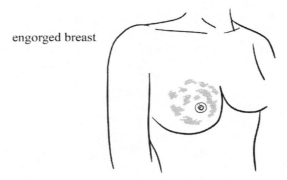

Engorged breasts are enlarged, firm and often red or darkened (in women of color).

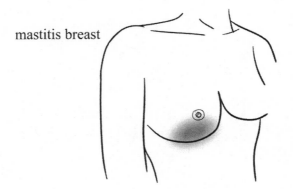

A breast with mastitis tends to be red, warm, and painful to the touch, especially with nursing.

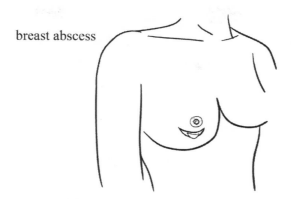

breast abscess

A breast abscess is usually characterized by a discrete area that is soft and fluid filled while the entire breast may be red or inflamed.

Things that can cause breast lumps when you are not pregnant can also occur during pregnancy, including any number of benign tumors of the breast as well as breast cancer. Rest assured, though, breast cancer is very rare during pregnancy.

TO DO LIST

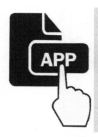

Make sure you check out the App section on how to do your Breast Self-Exam (BSE).

Breast Self-Exam (BSE): This section of the app has instructions on how to perform a BSE.

Why is it happening? The why, of course, depends upon the what.

1. **Enlargement of the breast glands:** Usually occurs as the hormones of pregnancy prepare the breasts for milk production.

2. **Blocked milk ducts:** Occur when the ducts that carry colostrum and milk from the gland to the nipple become blocked, causing the duct and gland to swell.

3. **Mastitis:** Is an infection of the breast tissue that usually occurs once the baby is actually breastfeeding. It is generally caused by bacteria from the baby's mouth infecting the breast tissue or infecting a blocked milk duct.

4. **Abscess:** Is a collection of pus that occurs in an infected milk gland.

5. **Benign lumps:** The most common of which is a *fibroadenoma* can actually be stimulated by the hormones of pregnancy.

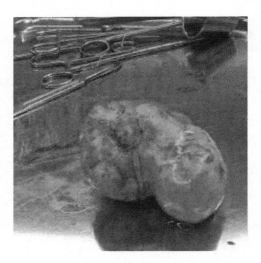

Fibroadenoma.

6. **Breast cancers:** Are rare in younger women, and are usually sporadic, meaning there is no prior family history.

Tell me more:

1. **Enlargement of the breast glands:** Usually causes generalized breast discomfort involving both breasts.

2. **Blocked milk duct:** Will cause swelling and discomfort with or without redness in an isolated area and usually affects only one breast.

3. **Mastitis:** Usually involves only one breast, and it is characterized by a swollen, red, painful breast that is warm to the touch and without a palpable lump.

4. **Abscess:** Usually is characterized by a large, soft mass in a red, warm breast.

5. **Benign lumps:** Most "other" lumps of the breast are benign, meaning they are non-cancerous. Their characteristics will ultimately depend on what condition you have.

6. **Breast cancer:** Can have a variety of symptoms or no symptoms at all. The lumps are usually firm and irregular in size and shape, they may move but are frequently difficult to move, and pain may or may not be present as may nipple discharge or bleeding. With breast cancer occurring in only 1 in 3,000 pregnancies, it is quite rare.

Can I treat this and will it get better? This, of course, depends upon the cause.

1. **Enlargement of the breast glands:** Cannot be treated but will usually improve after delivery or once you wean your baby.

2. **Blocked milk ducts:** Are generally treated with massage of the affected duct and the application of heat. With these measures, the symptoms usually resolve quickly.

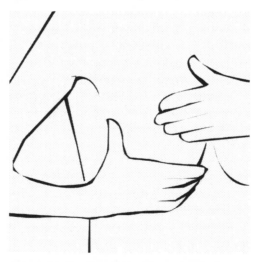

Massaging the blockage will help to dislodge it.

3. **Mastitis:** Requires oral antibiotics for treatment and usually improves soon after starting them.

4. **Abscess:** Requires antibiotics and frequently will also require drainage by your medical provider. With these measures, symptoms resolve quickly.

5. **Benign lumps:** Usually only require intervention if they are painful or getting larger. With intervention, improvement usually occurs quickly.

6. **Breast cancer:** Again, this is rare, but always requires treatment. Prognosis depends upon type and stage.

When should I call my provider? Anytime you notice a new mass or lump in your breast; you should notify your provider ASAP.

Old Wives Tale

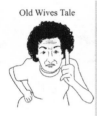

"All changes that you see in your breasts during pregnancy are always normal". Not true! While most breast changes during pregnancy are normal, you should always alert your provider to any atypical changes or changes that concern you.

Old Wives Tale

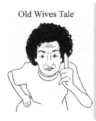

"Don't touch your breasts while pregnant!": Despite what you may have heard from an old wife, you should continue doing your breast self-exams even during pregnancy and lactation.

CHAPTER 11

PREGNANCY, THE BRAIN, AND NERVOUS SYSTEM

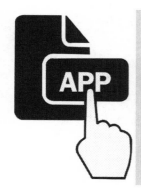

Don't forget to download the Everything Pregnancy app!

1). Who knew that pregnancy would literally be a headache?

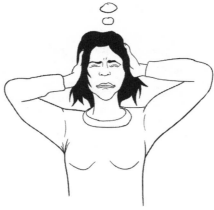

Headaches During Pregnancy:

Is this real, or am I imagining this? Headaches during pregnancy are very real and very common.

What is this? There are a lot of reasons to have headaches during pregnancy, including:

1. Physiologic headaches.

2. Allergy and sinus related headaches (see chapters 5 and 7).

3. Migraine headaches.

4. Musculoskeletal headaches.

5. Headaches due to hypertension/preeclampsia.

Why is it happening? The why depends upon the what:

> **Physiologic headaches:** This is the most common type of pregnancy-related headache, and it is caused by (yup, you guessed it) your hormones. Specifically, a hormone called progesterone causes your blood vessels to dilate, which in turn lowers your blood pressure, often resulting in dull headaches and dizziness. Not to be outdone, the hormone estrogen also contributes to physiologic pregnancy headaches.

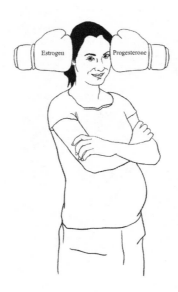

Migraine Headaches: Just like almost everything else that irks you during pregnancy, an increase in the frequency and intensity of migraines can in part be blamed on the hormonal changes of pregnancy (again primarily increasing levels of estrogen and progesterone). Many lucky mommies-to-be (two out of every three migraine sufferers), however, actually notice a decrease in migraine activity, so keep those fingers crossed.

Musculoskeletal Headaches: Guess what ladies, your mom was right! Posture is essential, and let's be honest; most people's posture sucks even without the excuse of pregnancy. Now strap a watermelon to your belly and an extra 35 pounds to your body, and what do you think happens? Bingo, your posture gets even worse.

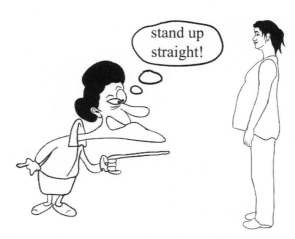

Headaches due to hypertension/preeclampsia: Are by far the most common, serious cause of headache during pregnancy. Preeclampsia is a hypertensive condition specific to pregnancy that affects most of the body's organ systems, including the brain. The effect of preeclampsia on the brain leads to frequent, and often severe, headaches.

Tell me more:

Physiologic headaches tend to start at the end of the first trimester (roughly 14 weeks) and become progressively worse until about 24 weeks. During this time, progesterone levels are increasing, which causes your blood pressure to decrease. Thankfully by 24 weeks, the progesterone level starts to fall, and your blood pressures begin to rise. Most mommies-to-be will notice that their headaches improve or completely resolve at this time.

Migraine Headaches: For those unfortunate sufferers who do notice an increase in migraine frequency or intensity during pregnancy, the peak intensity usually occurs during the end of the first trimester through the middle of the second trimester. Unlike physiologic headaches, however, migraine sufferers can experience headaches throughout pregnancy.

Headaches due to hypertension/preeclampsia are usually severe and are associated with other symptoms, including:

1. Visual changes (blurry vision, double vision, spots in the vision).
2. Pain in the middle or the upper right side of the abdomen.
3. Nausea and vomiting.
4. Extreme swelling of the legs and ankles and sometimes of the arms and hands.

Can I treat this? Well, of course, we would not be the Twin Docs if we didn't have some solutions for you, so here ya go:

TO DO LIST

Tip for daily living: Go for stronger flavors and try adding a touch of ginger.

Tips for Daily Living:

• *Stay well hydrated.*

• *Eat small, frequent meals, and always have a snack handy.*

• *Ice packs to the forehead and back of the neck.*

• *Massage and acupuncture.*

Physiologic headaches and migraine headaches: Physiologic headaches will usually resolve with time, often by the 24th week of pregnancy (during the 6th month). Physiologic headaches and migraines during pregnancy are treated similarly, and options include:

1. **Well hydrated:** Maintain adequate fluid hydration with at least 72 ounces of water daily or more.

2. **Well fed:** Keep your blood sugar steady by eating multiple smaller meals and snacks throughout the day.

3. **Lots of rest:** Finding a dark, quiet environment for a quick nap or to at least close your eyes for a few minutes will often do wonders.

4. **Ice packs** to the head and the base of the neck.

5. **Massage.** A good massage is a great way to relax the entire body while simultaneously treating a headache, so if you can't get a professional to do the heavy lifting, put your partner to work!

6. **Acupuncture.** Has been medically proven to reduce headache frequency and intensity.

7. **Caffeine:** Check with your provider first, but for most pregnant women, up to 12 ounces of caffeine daily is okay. A bit of caffeine at the start of a headache can frequently prevent the headache from getting worse.

8. **Tylenol:** Again, check with your provider before starting any new medication, however, acetaminophen/ Tylenol is generally safe for use during pregnancy (up

to 1,000mg every 8 hours) and much like caffeine, when used at the initial sign of a headache, it tends to work better.

9. **For migraine sufferers, many medications that could be used before pregnancy can also be used during pregnancy**, including beta-blockers and Imitrex, to reduce headache frequency and intensity. As always, consult with your provider before starting a new medication or resuming an old medication during pregnancy.

Posture-related headaches: These can generally be relieved with better posture. Simple, right? Well, not necessarily, especially during pregnancy, which is why we recommend using a *belly belt*. The belly belt lifts the pregnant uterus while supporting the lower back and returning the center of gravity closer to its usual pre-pregnancy location. Other things that help posture-related headaches include ice packs to the neck and head, massage, acupuncture, and acetaminophen (Tylenol), but as always, make sure you speak with your provider first.

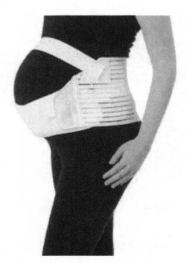

Pregnancy belt.

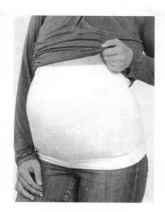

Pregnancy band.

Hypertension/Pre-Eclampsia: The only treatment for Pre-eclampsia is delivery. The timing of delivery is based upon how severe your blood pressure readings are and how far along you are in your pregnancy. There are things that your doctor can do to treat your headache related to hypertension/pre-eclampsia, and this is not something that should be treated at home. For more information, refer to the section in Chapter 26 on Pre-Eclampsia and Gestational Hypertension.

Will this get better?

Physiologic headaches tend to resolve by the end of the second trimester (around 24 weeks), so take some of the steps above, and just bide your time.

Migraine Headaches: Many sufferers notice that their headaches do start to improve (both in terms of frequency and intensity) as they reach the end of the second trimester. Some unlucky, however, will experience migraines throughout their pregnancies.

Posture-related headaches: Untreated, they will improve after delivery once your center of gravity and posture return to their pre-pregnancy states. However, if your posture sucked before pregnancy, it will likely continue to suck after pregnancy, and headaches may continue.

Preeclampsia: Because preeclampsia is a condition of pregnancy, once delivery occurs, the symptoms do tend to rapidly dissipate, though it can take up to 12 weeks for all symptoms to completely resolve.

When should I call my provider? Reach out to your provider any time you have a question or concern. Definite reasons to call your provider include:

1. Sudden onset of a severe headache.
2. A headache that will not go away despite interventions.
3. Frequent headaches, especially if they don't respond to Tylenol.
4. Headaches associated with visual changes (seeing spots, double vision, seeing stars).
5. Headaches associated with abdominal pain.
6. Headaches with extreme swelling of the limbs.
7. Headaches associated with weakness, dizziness, or feeling faint.

TO DO LIST

Tips for Daily Living: If you are experiencing frequent headaches, be sure to go to the Headache Diary in the app, fill it out and share it with your provider.

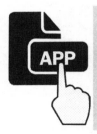

Headache Diary: Be sure to visit the Headache Diary in the app to log details of your headaches to share with your provider.

2). Is the world spinning, or is it just me?

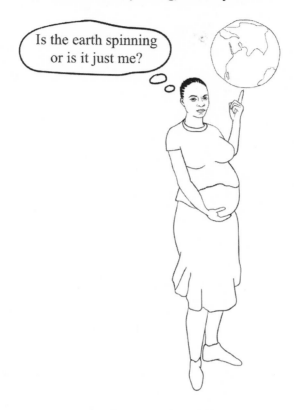

Dizziness During Pregnancy:

Is this real, or am I imagining this? Okay, clearly the world is spinning, but we get your point. Dizziness and lightheadedness during pregnancy are both extremely common.

What is this? We doctors haven't quite gotten around to giving this a super long, difficult to pronounce, scientific name, so let's just call it dizziness.

Why is it happening? There are many reasons women feel dizzy or faint during pregnancy, including:

1. Hormonal fluctuations: We can't get through a chapter without blaming this obvious culprit, but it's true folks. Progesterone causes your blood vessels to dilate so that they can carry more

oxygen-rich blood to your uterus and growing baby; that's a good thing. The problem is that those dilated blood vessels take less blood to your brain, causing dizziness and faintness; a not so good thing.

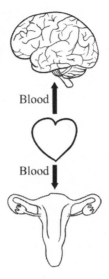

2. Your Growing Uterus: Yup, that growing baby factory puts a lot of pressure on the *inferior vena cava*, the large vein that brings blood from the lower parts of your body back to your heart. This reduction in blood flow again causes a reduction in the amount of blood reaching the brain, and *voila*, dizziness, and faintness result.

3. Blood Sugar Levels: It's not enough that your baby has taken your sense of comfort and wellbeing, but he or she also wants your sugar. Well not technically, but that sounded really dramatic, and we're all about the drama. Often during pregnancy, your blood sugar levels can be low because your growing baby and changing body need more sugar and because those doggone hormones are at it again, this time affecting sugar metabolism.

4. Dehydration: You need water and fluids more than ever when you are pregnant, and if you don't get them, your body has some pretty unpleasant ways of letting you know what you are missing.

214

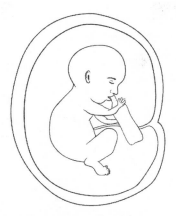

Be like the baby and stay well hydrated.

Tell me more: Dizziness and faintness are quite normal and are not dangerous conditions in and of themselves. The potential danger comes from the possible consequences of becoming dizzy or losing consciousness during certain activities like driving.

Can I treat this? Dizziness and faintness during pregnancy can't be eradicated, but they can be improved, and here are some things to try:

Prevention first!:

1. **Hydrate, hydrate, hydrate:** The more you hydrate, the higher your blood volume and the better your blood pressure.

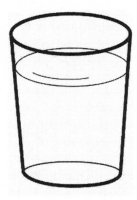

Don't be a stranger; get to know me.

2. **Eat, eat, eat:** Eat smaller meals more frequently to keep your blood sugar steady and adequate.

3. **Lay on your left side:** Once you are in the second trimester, lying on your back puts pressure from the uterus onto the inferior vena cava, reducing blood return to the heart.

4. **Avoid hot baths or showers, and avoid excessive heat in general:** Over-heating increases dizziness and increases the possibility of fainting.

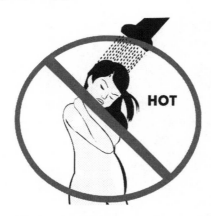

5. **Keep it in slow-mo:** When changing position (lying to sitting/standing or sitting to standing), go s l o w l y. Blood pressure typically drops when you change position, and this is exacerbated during pregnancy, so keep it slow and steady.

6. **Keep it movin':** Being sedentary reduces the return of blood from your legs to your heart. Staying mobile gets more blood pumping to your heart and brain.

7. **Granny support hoses:** Yup, Granny is on to something. Just like moving increases blood return from the lower extremities to your heart and brain, so do compression stockings, which minimize pooling of blood in the legs and feet.

8. **Wear loose clothing:** This helps the overall circulation of blood through the body and back to the heart and brain.

If Prevention fails, then there is always **Treatment:** If prevention fails, there are things that you can do when you're feeling dizzy or faint, including:

1. **Sit down with your head lowered**, or lay down without a pillow under your head.

2. **A cold compress** to the head and neck can help.

3. A few minutes of **deep breathing** can work wonders.

4. Open a window for **fresh air**, or sit under a fan.

5. **Loosen your clothing** (belt and pants, shirt or jacket).

6. **A quick burst of sugar**, like a small, soft candy, once you are sure you are not going to faint can help.

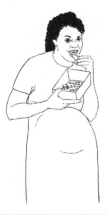

TO DO LIST

Tip for daily living: Go for stronger flavors and try adding a touch of ginger.

Tips for Daily Living:

TO DO LIST

• Borrow your grandma's support hose.

• When in bed, stay on your left side.

• Stay watered. Hydrate, hydrate, hydrate!

• Always keep a snack handy and eat throughout the day.

• Avoid excessive heat.

Will this get better? Dizziness and faintness tend to be at their worst during the first and second trimesters, improving during the third trimester, and resolving within a few weeks of delivery.

When should I call my provider? You should reach out to your provider if your dizziness or faintness:

1. Does not resolve after a few minutes.

2. Is associated with headaches that do not resolve.

3. Is associated with a severe headache.

4. Is associated with chest pain or loss of consciousness.

5. Is debilitating.

3). Should I be passing out?

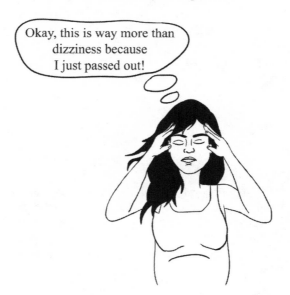

Fainting During Pregnancy:

Is this real, or am I imagining this? For many mommies-to-be, the dizziness and faint feeling that is so common during pregnancy can actually result in a loss of consciousness (fainting).

What is this? The technical name for loss of consciousness is *syncope*.

Why is it happening? The most common cause of syncope during pregnancy is the lowered blood pressure and relatively decreased blood flow to the brain that we already discussed earlier in this chapter. There are other rare, but potentially serious, causes of syncope as well including:

1. High blood pressure/preeclampsia.

2. Dehydration.

3. Heart conditions.

4. Seizures.

5. Neurological Causes.

6. Ectopic pregnancy (a pregnancy in the fallopian tubes instead of the uterus).

Tell me more: Thankfully, all of those way more frightening causes of syncope are infrequent, with the exception of dehydration, and most syncopal episodes are related to the hormonal and physical changes of pregnancy. Having said that, no incident of syncope should be ignored, ever!

Can I treat this? The best treatment for syncope is prevention. **Prevention involves**:

1. Hydration.

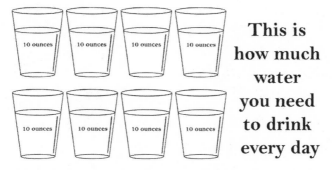

This is how much water you need to drink every day

2. Smaller, more frequent meals with a bit of sugar.

3. Avoiding extreme heat.

4. Avoiding sudden movements or prolonged inactivity.

5. Wearing loose clothing.

6. Whenever you are lying down, lay on your left side.

7. If you have had a past syncopal episode, do not drive until your provider says that it is okay; consider sitting in the shower (get a shower chair), and definitely avoid heights.

If you have a syncopal episode, the first thing to do is seek immediate medical attention:

1. Someone should call 911 if consciousness is not regained.

2. Call 911 or have someone take you to the nearest emergency care location if consciousness does return.

TO DO LIST

TO DO

Tips for Daily Living:

- *Chug-a-Lug: Drink 72 ounces of water or more per day.*

- *Always have a snack handy, and eat smaller more frequent meals.*

- *Avoid extreme heat.*

- *Stay mobile, and wear loose clothing.*

Will this get better? If you have multiple episodes of syncope during pregnancy, you and your provider should investigate other possible causes. Syncope strictly related to the physical and hormonal changes of pregnancy will usually improve within weeks of delivery. If the symptoms do not improve after delivery, you and your provider should search for other potential causes.

When should I call my provider? You should call your provider immediately if you experience any of the following:

1. Syncope/passing out.

2. Seizure-like activity.

3. Head or abdominal trauma.

4. A severe headache or visual changes.

5. Abdominal pain or vaginal bleeding.

6. Extreme weakness or dizziness.

CHAPTER 12

MUSCLES, JOINTS AND PREGNANCY

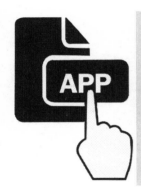

Don't forget to download the Everything Pregnancy app!

1). Why do all of my joints ache?

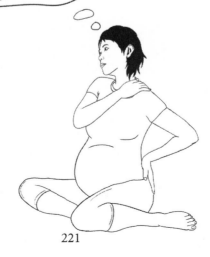

All of my joints seem to ache. Am I becoming a mother or a grandmother?

Joint Pain During Pregnancy:

Is this real, or am I imagining this? Joint aches and pains during pregnancy are very real. The pregnant woman who finishes pregnancy without experiencing joint discomfort is the rare exception.

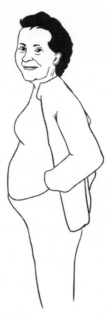

What is this? The technical name for joint pain is *arthralgia*.

Why is it happening? Pregnancy-associated arthralgia is caused by the many anatomical changes that occur during pregnancy. Here are a few of those changes:

1. Weight gain: Weight gain and pregnancy go together like peas and carrots, and yes, life is like a box of chocolates. Anytime you gain weight; you put extra pressure on the larger, weight-bearing joints, namely the spine, hips, knees, and ankles. This weight gain naturally causes joint pain and discomfort.

2. Fluid retention: Pregnant women retain roughly 50% more fluid than non-pregnant women, and all of this fluid has to go somewhere. Some of those places are the larger joints, think knees and ankles, as well as the smaller joints like the fingers and toes. This added pressure again causes joint pain and discomfort.

3. Hormonal changes: Yup, those dang hormones are back again! Specifically, progesterone and relaxin, both of which are elevated during pregnancy. These two hormones cause joints to become softer and laxer, changes that serve a purpose, namely allowing the pelvis to widen to accommodate the growing uterus and to further relax during delivery. These softer, looser joints, however, frequently cause joint pain and a feeling that the joints are more flexible than usual.

Tell me more: There are other less common causes of joint pain that are not specific to pregnancy, including:

1. Hypothyroidism: Which is an underactive thyroid gland.

2. Arthritis: Which is inflammation of the joints.

3. Autoimmune diseases: Like Lupus and rheumatoid arthritis, which frequently have joint pain and swelling as a symptom.

Can I treat this? While joint pain and discomfort usually can't be wholly eradicated during pregnancy, some things can be done to make those aching joints feel a lot better, including:

1. **Apply cold:** Cold compresses, or even frozen vegetables applied to the joints can reduce the swelling and inflammation that cause joint pain.

2. **Mechanical support:** A significant factor in joint pain is the hyper-flexibility of the pregnant joints, and this is where support comes in. Knee, ankle, and elbow braces can be easily purchased at a local pharmacy or medical supply store, and they provide some much-needed support.

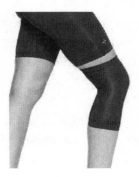

Knee brace.

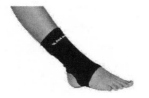

Ankle brace.

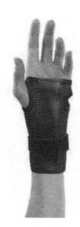

Wrist brace.

3. **Belly belt or belly band:** These devices, designed specifically for pregnant women, elevate the uterus, taking pressure of off the hips and lower extremity joints.

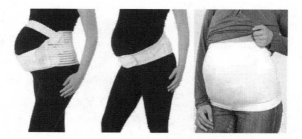

4. **Elevate your legs:** Elevating your legs will reduce excess fluid buildup, which will, in turn, reduce joint pain.

5. **Sleeping position**: It is always best to sleep on your left side, especially during the third trimester of pregnancy. Sleeping on

the left side will reduce the pressure placed by the uterus on the hips and lower extremities.

6. **Massage:** A good prenatal massage will do wonders for your aching muscles and joints, not to mention your sense of wellbeing.

7. **Acupuncture:** This is another good option for relieving joint pain and a myriad of other pregnancy-related aches, pains, and discomforts.

8. **Pain Relievers:** When all else fails, Acetaminophen will reduce pain and inflammation in the muscles and joints. Just remember, Acetaminophen is the only safe pain reliever to take during pregnancy.

9. **Proper footwear:** Keep it comfortable and practical with flat, wider shoes. High heels and other uncomfortable shoes increase foot and ankle pain as well as pain in the higher joints (knees, hips, and spine).

TO DO LIST

Tips for Daily Living:

#1. Support stockings, braces and belts/bands.

#2. Ice and elevation.

#3. Massage and acupuncture.

Will this get better? Thankfully joint discomfort associated with pregnancy does eventually subside though it can take up to 12 weeks after delivery for those hormones and their effects to completely go away. If chronic, non-pregnancy related conditions cause your joint discomfort, it may improve after birth, but will likely not go away completely.

When should I call my provider? Call your provider if you experience:

1. A sudden increase in the amount of joint pain.

2. Extreme swelling, redness, and/or pain in one or both extremities can be signs of a blood clot or DVT (deep vein thrombosis).

3. Muscle weakness.

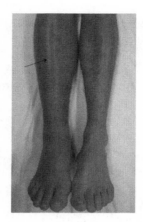

Signs of DVT (deep vein thrombosis) include leg swelling, redness, pain, and warmth.

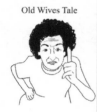

Old Wives Tale

"Of course you have swelling, you are pregnant!": *Not all swelling during pregnancy is normal. If you notice swelling that is more pronounced on one side, especially if it is associated with redness, pain, and/or warmth of the affected limb, you should contact your provider ASAP.*

2). Why do my legs cramp so much, especially at night?

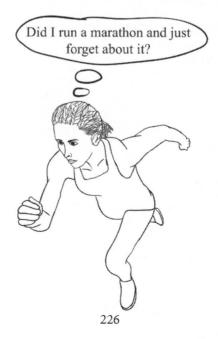

Did I run a marathon and just forget about it?

Muscle Cramps and Charlie Horses During Pregnancy:

Is this real, or am I imagining this? You guessed it, this is real, and you are not imagining this.

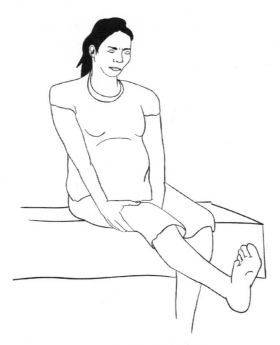

What is this? Muscle cramps and Charlie horses are simply *muscle spasms*.

Why is it happening? A muscle spasm occurs when a muscle involuntarily contracts, causing painful cramping and a twitching sensation. While quite common, there are a few reasons that muscle spasms occur more frequently during pregnancy, including:

1. Dehydration: Hydration during pregnancy is crucial for a variety of reasons. In the case of muscle spasms, dehydration can cause an electrolyte imbalance, which causes the muscles to spasms (see below).

2. Electrolyte imbalance: While dehydration can cause electrolyte imbalances, electrolytes can also be imbalanced in properly hydrated people. Certain electrolytes, namely *Potassium, Calcium,* and *Magnesium*, play an essential role in the

conduction of nerve impulses from your brain to your muscles. When these electrolyte levels are out of balance, the electrical impulses start to misfire, and you get a muscle spasm.

3. Excessive muscle use: No matter what your level of activity during pregnancy, the sheer work of lugging this extra life around with you 24-7 puts additional stress and strain on your muscles making them more prone to muscle spasms.

4. Poor flexibility: Your muscles are made to stretch and contract, and if you don't stretch them out appropriately, they will contract more than normal, which results in muscle spasms.

Tell me more: More than half of pregnant women experience at least occasional muscle spasms, and most pregnant women who experience them have them frequently. Muscle spasms tend to occur more frequently at night, and while they can involve any muscle, they most often occur in the lower extremities (calf muscles).

Can I treat this? When it comes to muscle spasms, an ounce of prevention is definitely worth a pound of cure. The best way to treat a muscle spasm is to avoid getting one in the first place. **So, how can you avoid getting muscle spasms?**

1. **Adequate hydration:** Drink 72-80 ounces of water per day.

2. **Take a prenatal vitamin** that contains potassium, calcium, and magnesium.

3. Consider eating **foods rich in potassium** like bananas and kiwis.

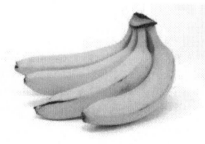 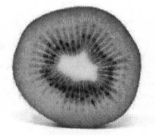

4. **Stretch your muscles a few times a day** to increase flexibility and reduce the likelihood of spasms.

PREGNANCY STRETCHES

01. Shoulder Circle

While seated or standing, rotate your shoulders backwards and down in the largest circle you can make

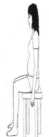

02. Chest Stretch

Place both hands at shoulder height and step forward with your right leg to apply pressure. Hold for 30 seconds. Repeat with left

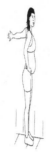

03. Hamstring Stretch

Place one leg on an elevated surface, with your back straight, bend from the waist. Hold and repeat 5-10 times

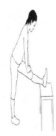

04. Neck Stretch

Tip your head to one side and use the arm on that side to pull your head towards your shoulder stretching your neck

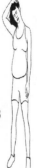

05. Labor Squat

This is just what is sound like Balance your body by steadying yourself with a counter, table or piece of furniture and squat for one minute at a time 10 times a day

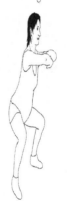

06. Pelvic Rocking

While on hands and knees, tilt your pelvis by contracting your deep abdominal muscles and pulling your belly button towards your spine. The movement is very small and your back should remain relatively flat.

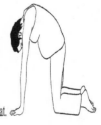

If you feel pain attempting these exercises, call your medical provider.

If you do experience muscle spasms, there are things that you can do at the moment to make them better, including:

1. **Massage:** Massage the involved muscle and the surrounding muscles during and after the spasm.

2. **Apply ice** during a spasm, especially as you massage the muscle.

3. *Stretch the involved muscle during a spasm.*

4. **Tylenol** can help with the post-spasm soreness.

Will this get better? Pregnancy-related muscle spasms are just that, pregnancy-related, and they usually go away within weeks of delivery.

When should I call my provider? If your muscle spasms are:

1. Severe and not improved by any of the above measures.

2. Associated with severe leg swelling or redness, especially if it is restricted to only one side. If this occurs, you should inform your provider ASAP.

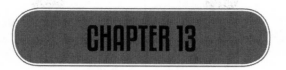

PREGNANCY AND THE URINARY TRACT

1). I feel like I am always in the bathroom!

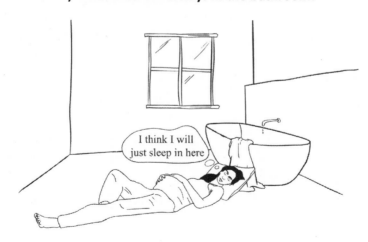

Pregnancy and Urinary Frequency:

Is this real, or am I imagining this? Urinary frequency during pregnancy is definitely real. At some point, almost every pregnant woman will feel like she is spending more time in the bathroom than any other room in the house.

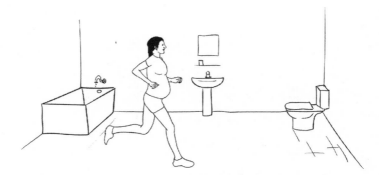

What is this? The technical term for this condition is *urinary frequency,* and it occurs when you are urinating more frequently than you usually do. In some cases, you can actually have *polyuria,* which is when you urinate more than 2.5 liters a day (if you really want to measure it out).

Why is it happening? You've probably guessed it— the pregnancy hormones are largely to blame for your urinary woes and specifically the hormone hCG. During pregnancy, your kidneys go into over-drive because hCG increases blood flow to the kidneys. Add to this the fact that your body is retaining extra fluid anyway and *voila*, you have the perfect pee-pee storm. The thinking is that the kidneys work overtime to clear impurities from your system that could potentially be harmful to your developing bundle of joy, so there is a method to the madness.

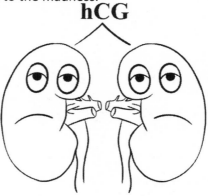

Tell me more: The excessive urination associated with pregnancy tends to be most pronounced during the first trimester (first 14 weeks of pregnancy) when the hCG levels are reaching their peak. While the frequency may improve a bit after the first trimester as hCG levels fall, compression from the growing uterus during the second and third trimesters will put more and more pressure on the bladder, reducing its ability to store urine which means you will still need to urinate more often.

Can I treat this? Because the urinary frequency is related to hormone levels and the growing uterus, there is no way to treat it. There are, however, things that you can do to reduce the need to spend your every waking hour in the bathroom, including:

1. **Empty your bladder more often:** This probably seems a bit counter-intuitive, but if you empty your bladder every 90-120 minutes, you will find that those instances of needing to go to the bathroom urgently will lessen.

2. **Empty your bladder more completely:** Once you finish urinating, lean slightly forward to get those last few drops out of the bladder.

3. **Hydrate, hydrate, hydrate:** This may sound counter-intuitive again because the more you hydrate, the more you have to go to the bathroom, right? While this is true, adequate hydration is crucial to both a healthy pregnancy and your overall health, yet some mommies-to-be will reduce fluid intake to minimize urination, and this is absolutely the wrong thing to do. We always recommend getting 72-80 ounces of water daily!

4. **Reduce caffeine:** 10-12 ounces of caffeine daily during pregnancy is safe, but caffeine does increase your kidney's production of urine, which means more trips to the bathroom. And remember, sad as it is, chocolate is also a source of caffeine.

TO DO LIST

Tips for daily living:

#1). Empty your bladder every 1-2 hours.

#2). Increase water intake and lay off of the caffeine.

Will this get better? Like most pregnancy-related conditions, this too shall literally and figuratively pass. Most new moms notice a pretty significant improvement within hours of delivery, though it can take up to 12 weeks for your urinary pattern to return to its pre-pregnancy level.

When should I call my provider? You should contact your provider if you experience any of the following:

1. A substantial increase in urinary frequency over a short period of time.

2. Urine that is discolored or has a strong odor.

3. Painful urination.

4. Flank/back pain or fevers.

2). Why do I leak urine when I cough, sneeze, or lift?

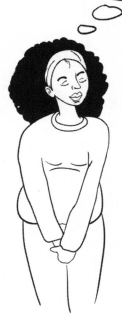

I laugh, I leak; I cough, I leak;
I stand up, I leak;
I skipped mommy and went
straight to grand mommy

Pregnancy and Leaking Urine:

Is this real, or am I imagining this? As if your life as a mommy-to-be isn't hard enough! Now you have to add leaking urine to the list. You are not imagining this, unfortunately. Just about every pregnant woman will experience leakage of urine at some point during her pregnancy.

What is this? The technical term for this leakage of urine is *urinary incontinence,* and specifically, in this case, *stress urinary incontinence.*

Why is it happening? As your bundle of joy grows, so does your uterus. Your growing uterus shares its neighborhood with the bladder, and she isn't always the best of neighbors as she encroaches more and more on the bladder's property. This uterine pressure both reduces how much urine your bladder can hold at any given time while simultaneously increasing bladder pressure, especially when you cough, sneeze, or even stand up. This results in leakage of urine.

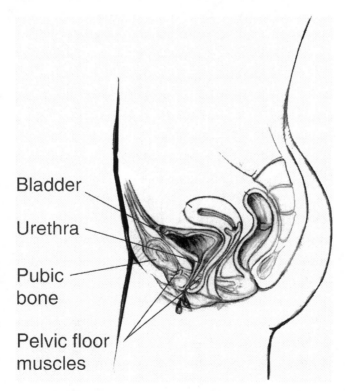

Bladder

Urethra

Pubic bone

Pelvic floor muscles

The bladder and the uterus live in the same neighborhood.

Tell me more: Not only does your growing uterus cause stress urinary incontinence (urine leaking with activity), but those pesky pregnancy hormones can also cause the bladder muscles to become over-active which causes leakage of urine. This type of incontinence is called *urge incontinence or overactive bladder.*

Can I treat this? While you can't generally "treat" urinary incontinence during pregnancy, there are things that you can do to reduce its frequency, including:

1. **Hydrate, hydrate, hydrate:** Hydration is vitally important during pregnancy, and you don't want to become dehydrated in an attempt to reduce urinary incontinence.

2. **Empty your bladder more frequently:** The more you empty your bladder, the less likely you are to leak urine with activity or when you have bladder muscle contractions.

3. **Reduce caffeine intake:** Caffeine increases urine production, which naturally increases the risk of incontinence. Caffeine has the added bonus of causing bladder muscle irritation, making it more likely to spasm.

4. **Reduce the intake of other things that can irritate the bladder muscles:** In addition to caffeine, tomato and citrus products can also irritate the bladder. Alcohol can as well, but alcohol use during pregnancy is an absolute no-no for other more important reasons.

5. **Wear a belly belt or belly band:** This lifts the uterus, relieving some of the pressure it places on the bladder.

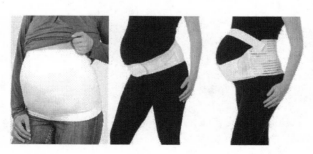

6. **Kegel exercises:** Kegels help strengthen the muscles in the pelvis that can be weakened by pregnancy and childbirth. A proper Kegel will cause the muscles of the vagina to contract as opposed to causing them to push downward.

7. **Keep your weight gain within the accepted range:** Weight gain during pregnancy is natural and expected, but excessive weight gain puts more unnecessary pressure on the bladder, increasing leakage.

8. **Sanitary Pads:** If all else fails, use a hypoallergenic pad to prevent soiling your clothing.

TO DO LIST

Tips for daily living:

#1). Keep yourself well hydrated.

#2). Empty your bladder more frequently.

#3). Wear a belly belt or belly band.

#4). Cut the caffeine.

Will this get better? The answer to this is yes and no. For most new moms, leakage of urine will definitely improve after delivery, but for a significant percentage of women, a certain degree of incontinence may remain after birth. Pregnancy and childbirth tend to cause a bit of damage to the *pelvic diaphragm,* which is a muscle that holds pelvic organs, including the uterus and bladder, in their proper place. Sometimes this damage may be irreversible. To add insult to injury, literally and figuratively, some woman will notice more stress urinary incontinence with each subsequent pregnancy and delivery. This is why Kegel exercises are a must during pregnancy as well as between pregnancies.

When should I call my provider? You should call your provider if you experience any of the following:

1. A sudden increase in urinary frequency.

2. Painful urination, especially if accompanied by back or flank pain and/or fevers.

3. Constant leakage of urine or fluid, in rare cases this could actually be amniotic fluid.

3). Do I really have another UTI?!

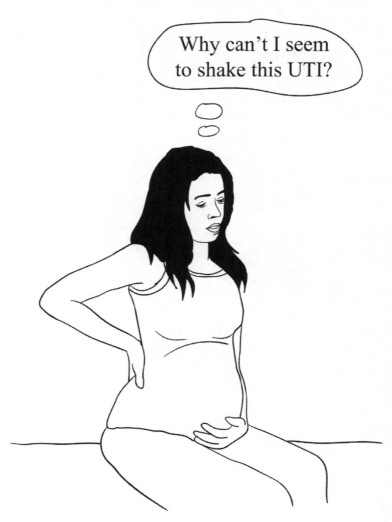

Frequent Urinary Tract Infections During Pregnancy:

Is this real, or am I imagining this? Many women do experience an increase in the frequency of UTIs (urinary tract infections) during pregnancy, so you are not imagining this.

What is this? Infections in the urinary tract occur in either the bladder, a condition known as *cystitis,* or the kidneys, a condition known as *pyelonephritis.*

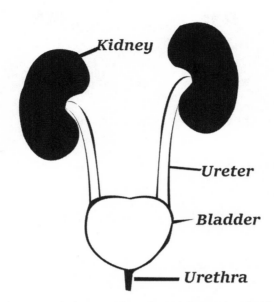

The ureters bring urine from the kidneys to the bladder.

Why is it happening? In general, women are more prone to developing UTIs because the shorter urethras allow bacteria from the external genitalia to get into the bladder more easily. Add to this the fact that we all leave some urine in our bladder after we urinate, and the fact that the growing uterus obstructs urine from flowing out of the bladder, and you have even more retained urine, which is a nice substance for bacteria to grow in. Sometimes these bacteria stay in the bladder, and sometimes they move up into the kidneys.

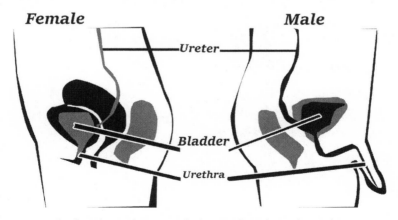

The female urethra is much shorter than the male urethra.
This is why women develop UTIs more frequently.

Tell me more:

Symptoms of cystitis (UTI in the bladder) include:

1. Increased frequency of urination even beyond the normal pregnancy-related increase.

2. Painful urination, often with a burning sensation.

3. Intense urge to urinate even though only a little urine is actually expelled.

4. Pain above the pubic bone where the bladder is located.

5. Cloudy or dark urine.

6. Strong urinary odor.

Symptoms of pyelonephritis (UTI in the kidney) include all the symptoms of cystitis plus:

1. Back or flank pain.

2. Fevers.

3. Chills.

4. Nausea and/or vomiting.

Interestingly, some UTIs have no symptoms, which is why your provider will likely be checking your urine at every office visit.

Can I treat this? UTIs can be both treated and prevented. When it comes to UTIs during pregnancy, an ounce of prevention is truly worth a pound of cure. Not only do UTIs cause physical discomfort, but left untreated (or treated too late) they can cause serious pregnancy complications, including preterm labor and pregnancy loss.

So first, what can you do **to reduce the risk of UTIs**:

1. **Hydrate, hydrate, hydrate, push the water:** The more water you drink, the more you flush your kidneys and bladder of potential bacteria.

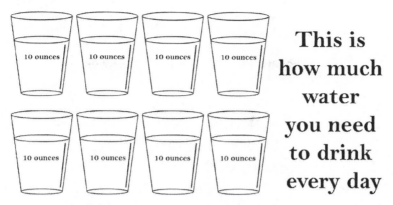

This is how much water you need to drink every day

2. **Empty your bladder frequently:** The longer urine remains in your bladder, the higher your risk of infection, so try to empty your bladder every 1-2 hours.

3. **Lean forward:** Once you are finished urinating, lean forward to squeeze that last little bit of urine out of your bladder.

4. **Drink Cranberry juice:** Cranberry Juice has anti-bacterial properties, and it should be a part of your UTI prevention regimen.

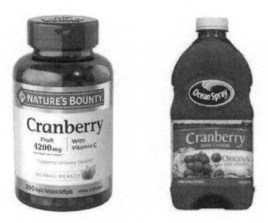

Cranberry juice works better than Cranberry tablets.

5. **Wear cotton underwear:** Cotton underwear reduces the number of bacteria on the external genitalia.

6. **Reduce your intake of sugar and caffeine:** Both sugar and caffeine increase the levels of bacteria in your bladder.

7. **Supplement with vitamin C:** 500mg daily will reduce your overall risk of infection.

8. **Empty your bladder before and after intercourse:** Intercourse helps the bacteria that typically live on the outside make their way into the bladder.

9. **Wipe from front to back:** Most of the bacteria that cause UTIs actually come from feces.

10. **Instead of wiping, consider blotting:** Blotting makes it less likely that you will push bacteria from the outside to the inside.

TO DO LIST

TO DO

Tips for daily living:

#1). Drink lots of water and cranberry juice.

#2). Empty your bladder frequently.

#3). Take vitamin C.

#4). Wear cotton underwear.

If you have symptoms of a UTI:

1. **Contact your provider immediately.** Early and appropriate treatment is crucial, especially with kidney infections.

2. **Antibiotics.** A short course of antibiotics, usually 3-7 days, will often be enough to treat a UTI. Most antibiotics that successfully treat UTIs are safe for use during pregnancy.

3. **Cranberry juice:** When it comes to prevention and treatment, cranberry juice has some beneficial properties, but it should be used in conjunction with antibiotics, not instead of them.

Will this get better? With proper treatment, most UTIs will get better. The increased incidence of UTIs that occurs during pregnancy usually does improve once your little bundle of joy enters the world and gets the heck off of your bladder.

When should I call my provider? If you suspect that you might have a UTI or if you have any of the symptoms listed above, you should contact your provider ASAP.

CHAPTER 14

PREGNANCY AND IT'S EFFECT ON YOUR ARMS AND HANDS

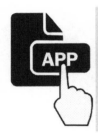

Don't forget to download the Everything Pregnancy app!

1). Either my hands are tingling, burning or I just can't feel them at all!

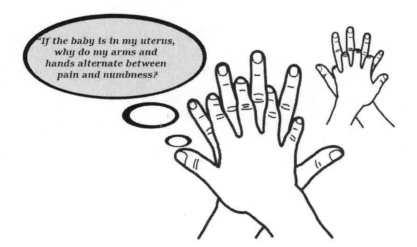

'If the baby is in my uterus, why do my arms and hands alternate between pain and numbness?

Carpal Tunnel Syndrome and Pregnancy:

Is this real, or am I imagining this? Yep, pain and numbness of the arms and hands are just another one of those fun things that come with the territory during pregnancy.

What is this? This is a phenomenon known as *carpal tunnel syndrome.*

Why is it happening? You've probably heard of carpal tunnel syndrome in people who do repetitive work with their hands like typists and phone operators. Carpal tunnel syndrome is caused by pressure on the *median nerve* as it passes through bones in the wrist known as the carpal tunnel. The pressure on the nerve causes pain, numbness, weakness, and tingling in the affected arm and hand.

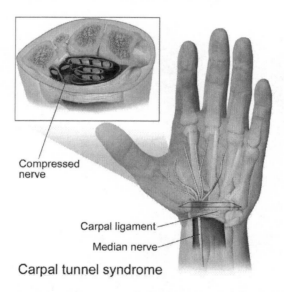

Compressed nerve

Carpal ligament

Median nerve

Carpal tunnel syndrome

The median nerve is surrounded by bones, blood vessels, and connective tissue. The extra fluid carried during pregnancy compresses the nerve causing the symptoms of carpal tunnel syndrome.

Tell me more: The extra fluid that all pregnant women retain causes the blood vessels to become engorged and leaky. The fluid, both inside and outside of the blood vessels, puts pressure on the median nerve. Symptoms of carpal tunnel syndrome are more common at night as the fluid that accumulated in the legs during the day distributes throughout the rest of the body, including the arms and hands. Carpal tunnel syndrome generally starts during the second trimester and continues throughout the pregnancy. For some women, carpal tunnel syndrome is just a minor annoyance; for others, it can be severe enough to make routine daily functions like eating, drinking, writing, typing, lifting, and carrying things difficult, if not impossible.

Can I treat this? Some things can be done to reduce the symptoms of carpal tunnel syndrome, including:

TO DO LIST

Tips for daily living:

#1). Do your stretching exercises at least three times a day.

#2). Use a wrist brace, especially when doing repetitive hand motions.

1. **Wearing a wrist brace:** Wrist braces can be found at any local pharmacy or medical supply store, and they work by reducing the amount of wrist movement, which in turn reduces pressure on the nerves in the carpal tunnel.

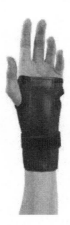

Wrist Brace.

2. **Application of ice or heat:** Start with ice because it reduces inflammation. If ice doesn't do the trick, heat works for some people.

3. **Acupuncture:** Many people report significant relief with acupuncture.

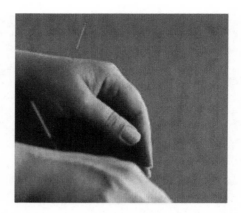

4. **Stretching Exercises**: Stretching the hands and wrists multiple times a day by flexing the hands up and down at the wrists reduces pressure on the median nerve.

Carpal Tunnel Stretching Exercises

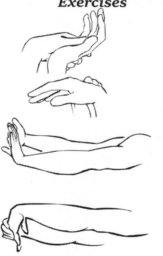

Starting with your wrist straight, flex, and extend the wrists multiple times.

TO DO LIST

Carpal tunnel stretching exercises: Be sure to check out that section of the app to see a video demonstrating carpal tunnel stretching exercises.

5. **Assume the proper position:** Keeping the wrists straight when working with the hands for prolonged periods of time will reduce pressure on the median nerve.

6. **Try not to sleep on your arms or hands.**

7. **Reduce salt intake:** More salt means more fluid retention, more fluid retention means more pressure on the median nerve.

8. **Tylenol as needed:** If all else fails, pain relievers can help.

Will this get better? For the vast majority of women, carpal tunnel syndrome (CTS) does improve soon after delivery. If CTS was an issue before pregnancy, it will usually get worse during pregnancy, but return to baseline after delivery. For the rare person for whom CTS remains a concern after delivery, there are treatment options available, including steroid injections and surgical intervention.

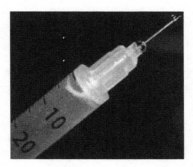

Steroid injections are quick, effective, and usually economical.

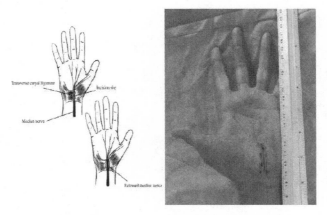

Small incisions are made over the wrist to access the nerve and reduce swelling and pressure on it.

When should I call my provider? You should contact your provider if you experience any of the following:

1. Pain so severe that you cannot function normally during the day or sleep at night.

2. Extreme arm swelling or sudden onset of swelling.

3. Significantly worsening pain, numbness, or weakness.

2). Why are my hands and face so swollen?

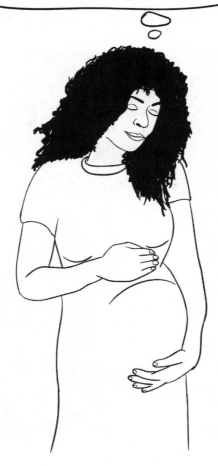

Swelling of the Upper Extremities During Pregnancy:

Is this real, or am I imagining this? You are not imagining this! While upper extremity swelling isn't as common as swelling of the lower extremities, many pregnant women do experience swelling in their hands and arms.

What is this? *Edema* is the technical term for fluid-induced swelling anywhere in the body, including the arms and hands.

Why is it happening? Much like edema in the lower extremities, swelling of the upper extremities is primarily related to the excess fluid that all pregnant women carry. Most women notice that if they do have upper extremity swelling, it tends to be most prominent in the morning because the excess fluids distribute throughout the body at night while you are lying flat.

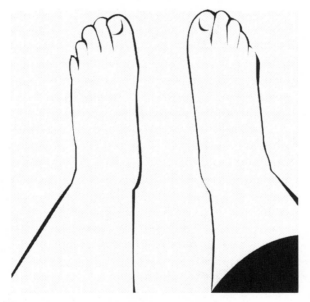

Typical edema of pregnancy starts at both ankles and can go all the way up to the knee. It can, at times, make its way to the upper extremities as well.

Tell me more: While swelling in the upper extremities is usually normal, upper extremity swelling can also be a sign of high blood pressure (*hypertension*) and specifically a condition known as *preeclampsia* (a type of hypertension during pregnancy).

Can I treat this? Upper extremity swelling is usually due to the excess fluid that all pregnant women have. While it cannot be "cured," there are things that can be done to reduce it:

TO DO LIST

Tips for daily living:

#1). Elevate your head during sleep.

#2). Avoid sleeping on your hands or arms.

#3). Drink dandelion tea

#4). Drink more water, use less salt.

1. **Sleep with a few pillows under your head** so that you are not entirely flat at night.

2. **Try not to sleep on your hands or arms.**

3. **Sleep on your left side.**

4. **Hydrate well.**

5. **Reduce your salt intake.**

6. **Dandelion tea** is known to reduce excess fluid retention and swelling.

7. **Wear loose clothing** for additional comfort.

8. **Take your rings off** before they become too tight to remove.

Will this get better? Much like swelling of the lower extremities, and just about every other condition of pregnancy, swelling of the upper extremities tends to dissipate within weeks of delivery.

When should I call my provider? You should reach out to your provider if you experience any of the following:

1. Swelling that comes on suddenly.

2. Swelling that is significantly more pronounced on only one side.

3. Swelling associated with symptoms of preeclampsia such as headaches, visual changes, abdominal pain, shortness of breath, or sudden weight gain.

CHAPTER 15

PREGNANCY AND YOUR LOWER EXTREMITIES

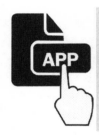

Don't forget to download the Everything Pregnancy app!

1). I never knew there were so many veins in my legs!

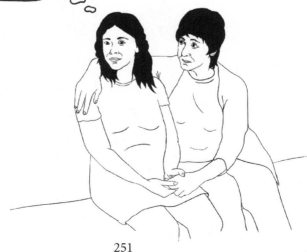

Pregnancy and Varicose Veins:

Is this real, or am I imagining this? We are genuinely sorry, but you are not imagining this. Varicose veins are frequently a very real part of pregnancy.

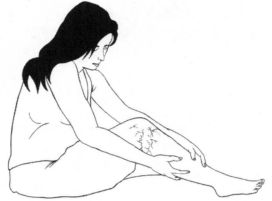

What is this? Varicose veins are swollen, enlarged veins that can usually be found anywhere below the waist but most frequently occur in the calves and legs.

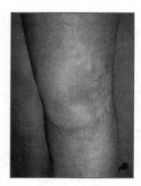

Varicose veins are frequently darker in people of color.

Why is it happening? Varicose veins occur during pregnancy for a multitude of reasons, including:

1. *The hormones of pregnancy*, including progesterone, cause the blood vessels to relax and dilate.

2. *The growing uterus* puts pressure on the vessels below the waist, causing them to become further engorged.

Tell me more: The woman who gets through pregnancy without varicose veins is definitely the exception and not the rule. While common, varicose veins are usually only an annoyance and not dangerous. Symptoms of varicose veins include:

1. Large, swollen, discolored veins.

2. Achy legs.

3. Itching or painful skin over the enlarged veins.

Can I treat this? Surgery is the only way to get rid of varicose veins completely, and this usually is not an option during pregnancy. There are, however, steps that can be taken to reduce the symptoms of varicose veins, including:

1. **Wear a belly belt or belly band:** These lift the uterus while providing support for the lower back. Lifting the uterus reduces pressure on the pelvic and lower extremity veins.

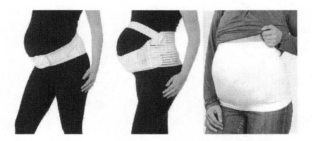

Different types of belly belts and belly bands.

2. **Wear pressure stockings or support hose:** These manually compress the varicose veins, reducing symptoms and vein size.

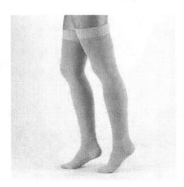

Support stockings.

3. **Elevate your legs:** This will fight the effects of gravity on your veins.

4. **Apply ice packs:** Ice packs will reduce the inflammation associated with varicose veins.

5. **Lay on your left side:** This will reduce the pressure that the uterus, which normally lies more on the right side, puts on the pelvic and lower extremity veins.

6. **Daily exercise:** Exercise improves blood return from the lower extremities to the heart.

7. **Minimize sitting,** and don't cross your legs when you do sit.

8. **Keep your weight gain within the desired range:** Extra weight leads to extra pressure, which makes varicose veins worse.

Will this get better? Varicose veins will usually resolve or at least improve after delivery. There are rare instances of varicose veins persisting after delivery, and these frequently require surgical intervention.

When should I call my provider? If you experience any of the following, contact your provider:

1. Pain in one or both legs.

2. Redness or warmth in one or both legs.

3. Skin discoloration.

4. Extreme swelling of one or both legs.

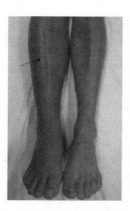

DVT. Notice the skin discoloration and the asymmetric swelling. This is indicative of a DVT, a potentially dangerous blood clot in the legs.

If you want to know about varicose veins of the external genitalia checkout chapter 9; if, however you just want to pretend that they don't exist, your secret is safe with us.

2). Just when I thought my legs couldn't get any bigger, they got bigger!

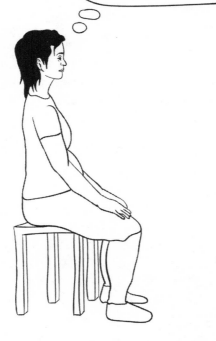

I never knew my legs
and ankles
could get this big!

Leg Swelling During Pregnancy (Edema):

Is this real, or am I imagining this? Like many of the other things we have talked about, swelling of the lower extremities is virtually a rite of pregnancy passage, so no, you are not imagining this.

What is this? The official name for this swelling is *edema*. Edema is a collection of fluid under the skin.

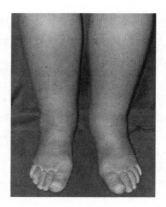

Leg edema.

Why is it happening? Edema is not restricted to pregnancy, but edema during pregnancy occurs for a few reasons:

1. *The pregnant body has roughly 50% more blood, and fluid* than the non-pregnant body, and the hormones of pregnancy cause the blood vessels to relax, which allows more of that fluid to escape.

2. *Pressure from the growing uterus* puts more pressure on the already leaky vessels in the lower extremities, which makes them leak even more.

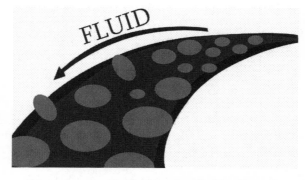

Edema is caused by fluid leaving the blood vessels,
going into the tissue below the skin.

3. *High blood pressure/preeclampsia:* While edema is quite normal during pregnancy, extreme or sudden onset of edema can be a sign of elevated blood pressure.

4. *Cardiomyopathy:* *Peripartum Cardiomyopathy* is a rare condition during pregnancy and the post-partum period in which the heart muscles do not pump effectively. A cough and shortness of breath usually accompany swelling in this case.

5. *Low potassium intake* can exacerbate swelling in the lower extremities.

6. *Excessive sodium intake* can also worsen swelling in the lower extremities.

7. *Exposure to extreme heat* is yet another possible cause for edema during pregnancy.

Tell me more: Interestingly, normal pregnancy associated edema tends to be slightly more pronounced on only one side of the body. Which side is dependent upon the side that the uterus deviates toward. For most women, this is the right side. The difference should only be slight, however.

Can I treat this? Edema usually can't be eradicated entirely, but some steps can be taken to reduce it, including:

TO DO LIST

Tips for daily living:

#1). Compress and elevate your legs.

#2). Hydrate, hydrate, hydrate!

#3). Lift with a belly belt or band.

1. **Belly belt/belly band:** These reduce pressure placed by the uterus on the vessels of the lower extremities.

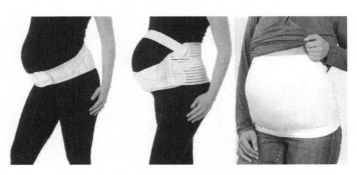

Different types of belly belts and belly bands.

2. **Pressure stockings/support hose:** While these do reduce edema, they are a temporary fix and don't solve the problem. Once you remove them, the swelling will return.

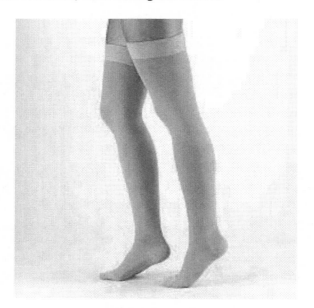

Support stockings.

3. **Elevate your legs when at rest:** When you sit or lay, let gravity reverse the effect that it has been having on your legs all day. Use pillows to keep your legs a few inches above your waist.

4. **Sleep on your left side:** This will reduce the pressure that your uterus places on the vessels of the pelvis and lower extremities.

5. **Maintain adequate fluid hydration:** 72-80 ounces of water daily, especially in excessive heat, will go a long way towards reducing edema.

6. **Reduce salt intake.** This one is pretty self-explanatory.

7. **Increase Potassium intake.** Usually 1-2 bananas a day is sufficient.

8. Break down and buy **wide width or larger shoes.** Style and fashion be damned!

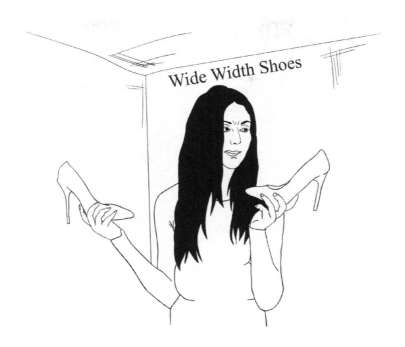

Will this get better? Edema will usually improve with the above measures, and it should completely resolve within weeks of delivery. If you find that despite doing the things above, your edema is not improving or if it doesn't improve after delivery, this could be a sign of something more serious, so let your provider know.

When should I call my provider? You should contact your provider if you experience any of the following:

1. Swelling that is extreme or sudden in onset.

2. Swelling that is significantly more pronounced on one side.

3. Swelling that is associated with headaches, visual changes, or abdominal pain.

4. Swelling that is associated with cough or shortness of breath.

3). Why do my legs cramp so much, especially at night?

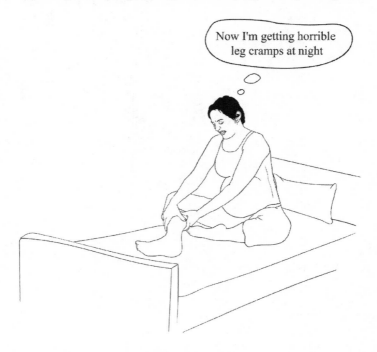

Leg Cramps and Pregnancy:

Is this real, or am I imagining this? Why, oh why, must pregnancy cause so many aches and pains? While we can't answer that cosmic question, we can explain why pregnancy-related leg cramps occur and confirm for you that you are not imagining this.

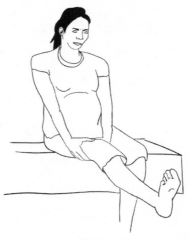

What is this? Most women start to notice leg cramps during the second trimester, and they usually continue throughout the rest of the pregnancy. These leg cramps are due to *muscle spasms.*

Why is it happening? While no one knows the exact reason for these muscle spasms, most theories blame a combination of pregnancy hormones, electrolyte imbalances (potassium, calcium, and magnesium), and fluid buildup in the legs.

Tell me more: These leg cramps occur more often at night (of course, I mean who needs a good night sleep during pregnancy anyway, right?), usually start in the calves, and then radiate up and down the legs.

Can I treat this? You likely won't be able to avoid this lovely side effect of pregnancy altogether, but there are some things you can do to reduce the frequency and intensity of these cramps, including:

TO DO LIST

Tips for daily living:

#1). Stretch often.

#2). Massage, massage, massage.

1. **Eat 1-2 bananas per day:** Bananas, being rich in potassium, will help to regulate your potassium levels, which will make your muscles much happier.

2. **Eat lots of yogurt:** Yogurt is rich in calcium, proper calcium levels also keep your muscles happy.

3. **Maintain adequate hydration:** This means drinking 72-80 ounces of water every day. Dehydration causes a multitude of problems during pregnancy, including electrolyte imbalances, which can lead to muscle cramps.

4. **Stretch:** Take two minutes every morning, afternoon, and evening to stretch the leg and calf muscles. This can be done by flexing the foot back and forth at the ankle.

Exercise to reduce leg cramping

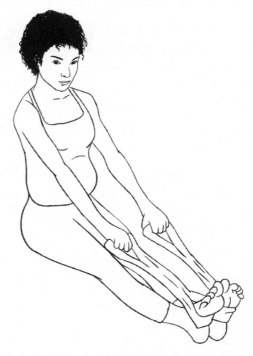

Keep your legs straight while flexing the ankles (pulling the balls of your feet towards your head).

5. **Massage the calves frequently**. Actually, this sounds like an excellent job for your partner. Let him or her share in a little bit of the fun!

When cramping occurs, there are things you can do to shorten the duration and associated pain:

1. **Gently massage** the area where the cramp originates. However, the key is to make sure that the massage is gentle, as a forceful massage can worsen the cramping.

2. **Stretch the calf muscles** by quickly flexing the foot at the ankle.

3. **Start with ice packs**, which reduce inflammation.

4. If ice doesn't work, **apply heat** to the affected area.

Will this get better? Like most pregnancy-related ills, leg cramping does rapidly improve after delivery.

When should I call my provider? You should contact your provider if:

1. Your leg cramping is severe enough to interfere with your ability to function normally during the day or sleep well at night.

2. The cramping is associated with extreme swelling, redness, or warmth of the affected leg.

3. You have weakness in the leg or problems walking on it.

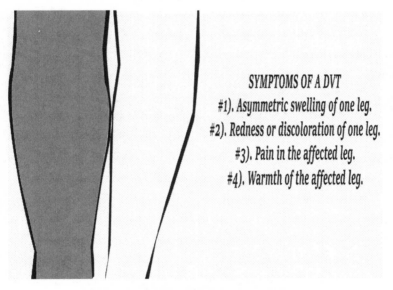

SYMPTOMS OF A DVT
#1). Asymmetric swelling of one leg.
#2). Redness or discoloration of one leg.
#3). Pain in the affected leg.
#4). Warmth of the affected leg.

A DVT (or deep vein thrombosis) is a potentially life-threatening blood clot that can occur in the legs.

CHAPTER 16

ENERGY DURING PREGNANCY

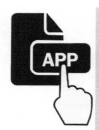

Don't forget to download the Everything Pregnancy app!

1). How am I supposed to get through the day when I can barely keep my eyes open?

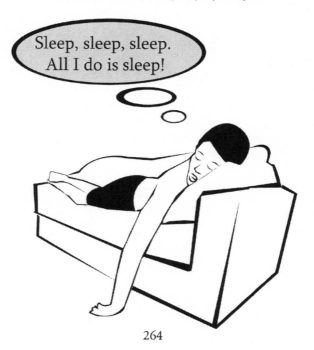

Pregnancy and Fatigue:

Is this real, or am I imagining this? Fatigue during pregnancy is very real, and it is one of the most common complaints that pregnant women have.

What is this? There are no fancy words this time; this is just good old-fashioned fatigue.

Why is it happening? When you think about what your body is doing, it really makes sense that pregnancy is exhausting. Your body is simultaneously supporting all of your needs and supporting the needs of another growing human being. This means that your overall metabolism is increased and your body is expending more energy at a time when its blood sugar levels and blood pressure are lower. Add to this the fact that the skyrocketing levels of the progesterone hormone make you sleepy anyway, and you have the perfect storm.

Tell me more: Luckily for the majority of mommies-to-be, fatigue is most pronounced during the first trimester (up to 14 weeks) and usually improves dramatically as you enter the second trimester. This second trimester of pregnancy is frequently called the *"golden period of pregnancy"* because many women experience an energy resurgence at the same time that their morning sickness is improving. Spoiler alert, fatigue will return during the third trimester, but it generally is not as severe as it is in the first trimester.

Can I treat this? No, there is nothing that will completely eradicate fatigue during pregnancy, but there are things that you can do to make it less of an issue:

1. **Nap often:** Your body knows what it needs, and the best treatment for pregnancy-related fatigue is to get a good nap. If this is your first baby, trust us, naps will soon be like solid gold, so enjoy them while you still can. If you work in the home, i.e. you have children who barely give you five minutes of privacy in the bathroom, or if you work outside of the home, a long nap is probably not realistic, but even taking a brief catnap (15-30 minutes at your desk on break or in your car) can make a world of difference.

Old Wives Tale

"Don't be lazy, if you sleep too much your baby will sleep too much": There is no such a thing as too much sleep. If you feel sleepy, listen to your body and take a nap anytime you are able to!

2. **Get some fresh air:** Consider opening a window or taking a brisk walk in the fresh air.

3. **Adjust your schedule:** You might be Superwoman, but even Superwoman needs a break. Give yourself a bit more time to get things done, and lighten your schedule as much as you can.

4. **Exercise:** It may seem counterintuitive, but 30 minutes of daily exercise will get the blood flowing, which helps to reduce fatigue.

5. **Make sure your diet is balanced:** Take your vitamins, hydrate, and eat energy-rich foods in smaller amounts throughout the

day. Consider a power snack that includes fruits for their natural sugars and nuts for their protein.

6. **Ask for help:** You likely didn't do this alone, so there is no reason that you should carry the entire burden. Certain anatomical constraints will prevent your partner from literally carrying some of the burdens, but feel free to divvy up the non-uterine burdens.

TO DO LIST

Tip for Daily Living:

#1. Nap, nap and nap again!

#2. Stay physically active and exercise.

#3. Don't be afraid to ask for help.

#4. Load up on proteins and natural sugars.

Will this get better? It definitely will. For many pregnant women, the extreme fatigue of the first trimester gives way to a burst of energy in the second trimester. Milder fatigue will likely return in the third trimester, and then it goes downhill from there…, as in waaaay downhill. Honestly, fatigue will be a way of life for the first six months or so after your little bundle of joy, aka "Nocturnal Hell Raiser," makes his or her big entrance. Just know that this too shall pass, and sleep will again be something that you enjoy.

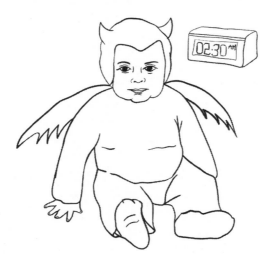

When should I call my provider? If you feel like your fatigue is so extreme that it is interfering with your ability to function normally during the day, you should contact your provider.

2). All of the sudden, I feel like I can do anything!

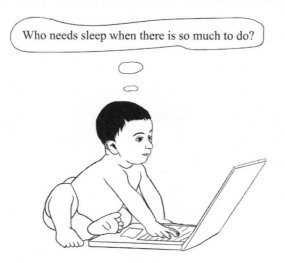

Who needs sleep when there is so much to do?

Sudden Burst of Energy During Pregnancy:

Is this real, or am I imagining this? Yup, this is real. Many pregnant women experience a burst of energy at the start of the second trimester, around 15 weeks, and again at the very end of pregnancy.

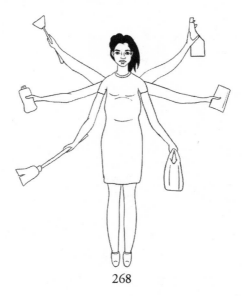

What is this? The burst of energy is frequently called *nesting*.

Why is it happening? The burst of energy that comes at the start of the second trimester is a result of the falling levels of the pregnancy hormone hCG and the plateauing levels of the hormone progesterone. No one really knows why the burst of energy at the very end of pregnancy happens, but anecdotally many people say that nesting may be a sign that labor is impending and it is your body's way of getting that "to do" list "to done." One can hope, right?

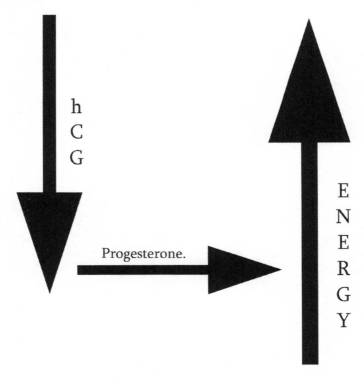

As your hormone levels fall or plateau, your energy will rise.

Tell me more: The resurgence of energy during the second trimester is part of what many people call *the golden period of pregnancy* when energy rebounds and nausea starts to wane. The burst of energy at the end of pregnancy is what people more frequently refer to as nesting, and many people believe this is your body's last hurrah, that final moment to get everything ready before the baby and the natural post-baby fatigue are a regular part of your daily "routine."

Can I treat this? Why would you want to?! Enjoy the energy while you have it!

Will this get better? We wouldn't call it "better," but the energy of the second trimester does start to wane at the end of the second trimester/start of the third trimester, and the nesting period at the end of pregnancy generally only lasts for a few days.

When should I call my provider? You should contact your provider if:

1. You feel like your energy resurgence is interfering with your ability to function normally during the day or sleep normally at night.

2. You have trouble staying focused or staying on task.

3. You experience racing thoughts.

4. You notice very fast or pressured (frenzied, rapid) speech.

CHAPTER 17

SEX, LIBIDO, AND PREGNANCY

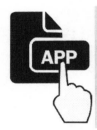

Don't forget to download the Everything Pregnancy app!

1). The idea of sex during pregnancy scares me!

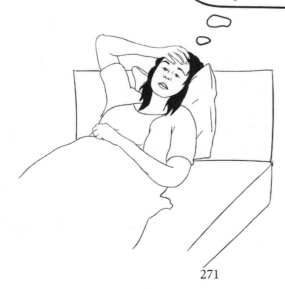

Who said that I can't have a headache for nine months?
I'm just not in the mood!

Sex During Pregnancy

Is this real, or am I imagining this? Many women, and men for that matter, have a fear that sex will harm their baby or somehow endanger their pregnancy. While this concern is very real, the fear in the vast majority of pregnancies is entirely unfounded.

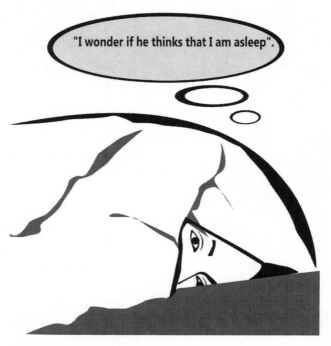

What is this? The technical name for fear of sex is *genophobia*, though many married couples would probably just call it the status quo.

Why is it happening? Many couples are concerned that the penis will hit the baby during intercourse. Others are concerned that having an orgasm will, in some way, be dangerous to the pregnancy or the baby. I hate to break it to all the fellas, but not even the most endowed penis can ever reach a baby in the uterus, and when it comes to orgasms, they are completely harmless for most uncomplicated pregnancies.

Tell me more: All of the changes that your body experiences during pregnancy have one goal, to protect and nurture your growing bundle of joy. This also holds true when it comes to sex during pregnancy. Here are the facts:

1. During sexual arousal, the average vagina lengthens to about 8 inches in length while the average erect penis is only about 5 inches in length. You can do the math there.

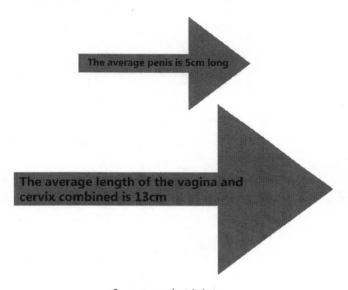

Sorry guys, but it is true.

2. The vagina (and penis during intercourse) are separated from the baby by many structures including the cervix, which can measure up to another 5cm in length, the mucus plug in the cervix, and the amniotic fluid that surrounds and cushions the baby.

3. Not only does having an orgasm not increase the likelihood of preterm labor, but some studies have actually found that women who have sex regularly in the second trimester have a lower chance of experiencing preterm labor compared to those who do not.

4. The baby may actually experience an improved sense of well-being from the endorphins that are released by mom during an orgasm. So, if not for you, do the baby a favor, and get busy!

Can I treat this? Fear of sex during pregnancy is common, but knowing the facts usually puts most couples at ease.

Old Wives Tale

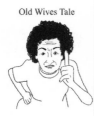

"Sex during pregnancy is a no-no": Not only can you have sex during pregnancy, but for the great majority of couples it is both a great physical release and a nice way to bond emotionally.

TO DO LIST

Tip for Daily Living: Pregnancy is not the time to skip foreplay. Foreplay will stimulate the lengthening of the vagina as well as the lubrication needed to make sex during pregnancy comfortable.

Will this get better? Even if knowing the facts hasn't quelled your fear, just remember all pregnancies do come to an end, and so too will yours. If you weren't afraid of sex before pregnancy, and if you are pregnant we're guessing you weren't, then you shouldn't be afraid of sex after pregnancy.

When should I call my provider? You should reach out to your medical provider if:

1. You have a higher risk pregnancy, including a history of prior or current preterm labor, previous preterm delivery, a cerclage in the cervix, multiple fetuses, rupture of membranes, hypertension, or placental issues.

2. This fear of sex is causing undue burden to you or causing problems in your relationship.

3. If you just need a bit more reassurance.

2). Why is sex so darn painful?!

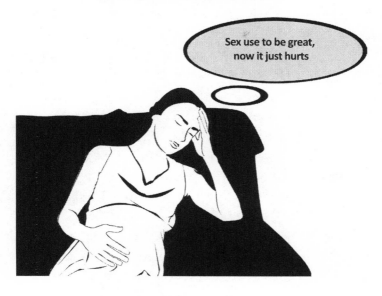

Painful Sex During Pregnancy:

Is this real, or am I imagining this? Many women do experience pain or discomfort with intercourse during pregnancy, so you are not imagining this.

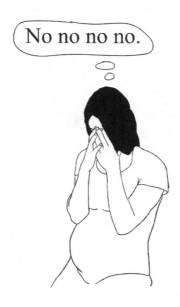

What is this? *Dyspareunia* is the technical name for painful intercourse.

Why is it happening? There are many reasons why intercourse may be painful during pregnancy, and they are generally caused by the normal anatomical changes that occur. Some of the more common causes of dyspareunia during pregnancy include:

1. Decreased vaginal lubrication: Most mommies-to-be will experience a decrease in vaginal lubrication during intercourse, which is somewhat ironic, given the overall increase in vaginal discharge that almost every pregnant woman will experience. Vaginal lubrication during intercourse is designed to reduce friction, and without it, sex will be uncomfortable or painful both during and after.

2. The growing uterus: As the uterus grows, it fills the entire pelvis. While the penis can't actually reach the baby, it can stimulate the back of the uterus through the vagina, and this uterine stimulation can cause pain, especially with deeper penetration.

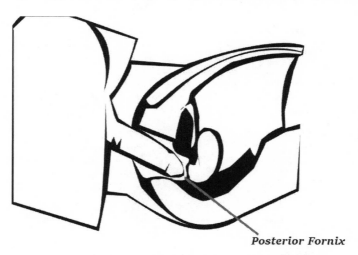

Posterior Fornix

The penis stimulating the posterior fornix (vagina behind the growing uterus) can cause pain or discomfort.

3. Infections: Vaginal and cervical infections (sexually transmitted and non-sexually transmitted) can also cause painful intercourse due to inflammation.

Tell me more: Some studies suggest that up to 50% of women will experience painful sex during pregnancy, so if this is you, you are definitely not alone. Fear not, there are things that you can do to alleviate or at least reduce some of the discomfort.

Can I treat this? While this is not something that can be treated per se, there are steps that you can take to reduce the pain associated with intercourse during pregnancy, including:

TO DO LIST

Tip for Daily Living:

#1. Don't be afraid to use water-based lubricants.

#2. Get creative with different positions.

1. **Use lubricants:** If decreased lubrication is causing painful intercourse, over-the-counter lubricants can be used safely during pregnancy. You should only use water-based lubricants since others can actually worsen the irritation.

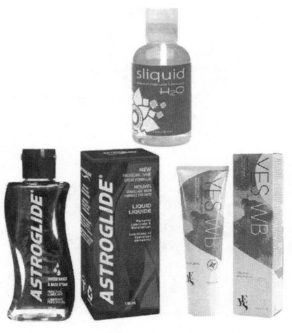

Various water-based personal lubricants.

2. **Change it up:** Position changes can reduce the depth of penile penetration, which should reduce pain. While we always encourage couples to enjoy the search for the positions that work best for them, frequently either "doggy style" (female on elbows and knees with the male partner entering from behind) or side-by-side work best.

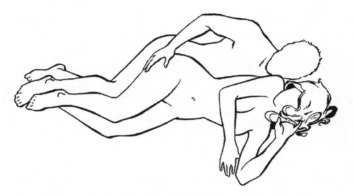

Side-by-side position reduces the depth of penetration.

Intercourse with the female mimicking the seated position again avoids the pregnant belly

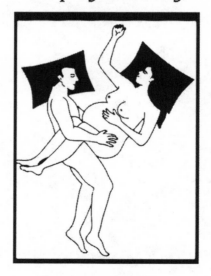

Female seated position.

3. **Infections (STDs and non-STDs) may or may not be associated with other symptoms,** so it is important to discuss this possibility with your provider. Infections should be treated ASAP during pregnancy because they increase the likelihood of preterm labor and delivery, and some can also cause harm to the baby if they are present at the time of delivery. There are medications that are completely safe for use during pregnancy to treat just about any potential vaginal or cervical infection.

Will this get better? Usually, painful intercourse during pregnancy will improve with the measures we discussed above. Even if you are not lucky enough to find some relief during pregnancy, like most other pregnancy-related ills, this too will pass. After delivery, once the anatomy and hormone levels return to their pre-pregnancy state, painful intercourse should no longer be an issue. If the cause of the discomfort was related to an infection, that pain should subside after the infection is treated.

When should I call my provider? As always, you should contact your provider any time you have questions or concerns. In particular, you should contact your provider if:

1. You have pain with intercourse that does not stop within 30 minutes of finishing.

2. You have bleeding or leakage of clear fluid.

3. You have signs of a possible infection, including abnormal or foul-smelling discharge, vaginal itching, or vaginal burning.

3). Why does it feel like my vagina is swollen?

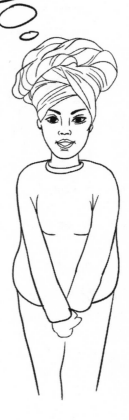

I feel like my nether-regions
are constantly
swollen and engorged...
not that I'm necessarily complaining

Pregnancy and Genital Engorgement:

Is this real, or am I imagining this? Genital engorgement during pregnancy is very real, and many mommies-to-be will experience the sensation of swelling, pressure, warmth, and/or fullness in the genital region.

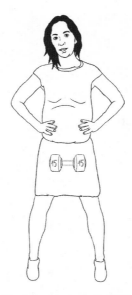

What is this? These sensations are collectively known as *genital engorgement.*

Why is it happening? Certainly, by now, you know that growing a baby takes a lot of hard work, and you also know that most of this work takes place between your belly button and your knees. While blood flow increases body-wide, most of that extra blood flow is directed to your uterus and vagina. This increased blood flow, combined with the pressure exerted by the growing uterus, leads to the sensation of genital pressure, fullness, warmth, and even throbbing and pulsations.

Tell me more: All that extra blood flow to the uterus and genitals brings oxygen and nutrients to your growing baby while carrying waste away from the baby. So, how much extra blood-flow is required to support your little bundle of joy? Would you believe a half liter of blood is flowing to your uterus every minute?! To put that into perspective, that is about 10% of your total blood volume going to your uterus each and every minute!

Can I treat this? Some women report that this sensation is not entirely unpleasant, but many mommies-to-be could definitely do without it. If it is bothersome, there are some things that you can do to reduce the sensation of genital engorgement including:

Tip for Daily Living:

#1. Position, position, position. Lift the uterus, recline when able, and lay on your left side.

1. **Belly belt or belly band:** Wearing a belly belt or belly band elevates the uterus, which in turn relieves pressure and engorgement.

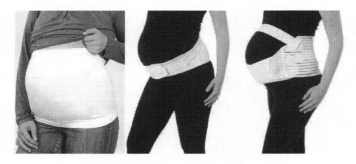

Belly band and belly belt.

2. **Ice packs***:* Cold causes blood vessels to constrict, a process called *vasoconstriction,* which by reducing blood flow reduces the symptoms of genital engorgement.

3. **Positional changes:** Gravity exacerbates the sensations associated with genital engorgement, so consider taking a seat or even reclining whenever possible. When in bed, lying on the left side reduces genital engorgement by tilting the uterus off of the pelvic vessels.

4. **Pelvic Support Garment:** Pelvic support garments are akin to a belly belt for south of the border. There are pelvic support garments designed specifically for pelvic prolapse, an issue seen usually in post-menopausal women, as well as for pelvic pressure, genital swelling, and vulvar varicose veins. These pelvic support garments are generally quite beneficial for mommies-to-be experiencing genital engorgement symptoms as well.

Will this get better? Of course, it will improve once that bowling ball that you lovingly call your bundle of joy makes his or her exit. Because genital engorgement is the result of hormonal fluctuations and anatomical changes, the symptoms will improve upon delivery, though it can take up to 12 weeks for complete resolution.

When should I call my provider? You should consider calling your provider if you experience any of the following:

1. A sudden, unrelenting increase in pressure.

2. Cramping and/or contractions.

3. Spotting or bleeding.

4. Leakage of fluid from the vagina or excessive vaginal discharge.

5. A decrease in fetal movement.

4). What is wrong with me; all I want to do is have sex!

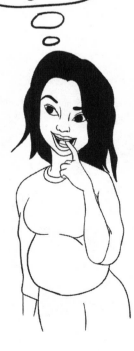

I feel like an adolescent boy, I can't get enough sex!

Increased Libido During Pregnancy:

Is this real, or am I imagining this? You're not imagining this. You are just horny, and many mommies-to-be are just as horny as you are.

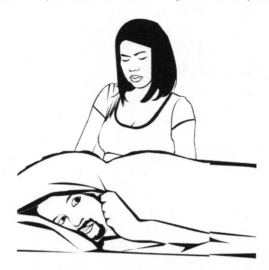

What is this? There is no scientific term for a pregnancy-related increase in libido, so we are just going to stick with the time-honored term *horny*.

Why is it happening? Increased libido during pregnancy can occur for a few reasons, including:

1. Fluctuating hormones, especially during the first trimester: For many women, this increase in hormones results in an increased desire for both sex and intimacy.

2. Genital Engorgement: For some women, the sensation of pelvic fullness and engorgement causes increased baseline arousal.

3. Not having to worry about getting pregnant: For many mommies-to-be, this can be quite the aphrodisiac. Pregnancy is the first time in the sexual lives of many women that they have been able to be sexually active without having that concern for pregnancy somewhere in their mind.

Tell me more: This increased libido is usually most pronounced in the first trimester and the early part of the second trimester when the hormonal fluctuations are at their greatest. While there may be a reduction in the third trimester, for many women this increase in libido will continue through the end of the pregnancy.

Old Wives Tale

"You can't have sex during pregnancy!": Not only is it okay to have sex during a low risk pregnancy, it actually has physical and emotional benefits for mom, partner and baby, so get busy!

Can I treat this? No, and why would you want to? Unless you have a high-risk pregnancy and have been advised by your provider against it, intercourse during pregnancy is both physically and emotionally healthy. Physically, sex is a great aerobic workout (if done properly ☺); it promotes more sound sleep; it increases the bond between partners (which can sometimes be strained by pregnancy), and studies have shown that it can even result in less preterm labor and preterm birth.

TO DO LIST

TO DO

Tip for Daily Living: There is nothing wrong with self-pleasuring during pregnancy. If either you or your partner do not feel comfortable with vaginal intercourse, or vaginal intercourse is not an option for other reasons, masturbation is okay as long as internal devices are not used and your provider says it is okay.

Will this get better/change? For some women, this increase in libido tends to wane a bit as the second trimester progresses. Unfortunately for a host of reasons that we will address in the *Everything Post-Partum* book, many women do have a pretty pronounced decline in libido after delivery (dropping hormones, sleeplessness, depression, etc.).

When should I call my provider? If you ever have a question or concern, you should contact your provider.

5). I don't care if I never have sex again!

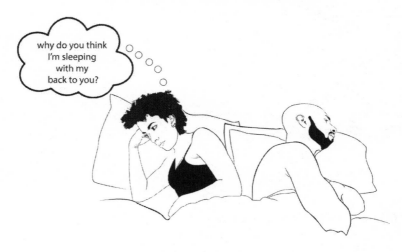

Low Libido During Pregnancy:

Is this real, or am I imagining this? You are not imagining this. Just like some women can experience a heightened libido during pregnancy, others will experience a lower libido.

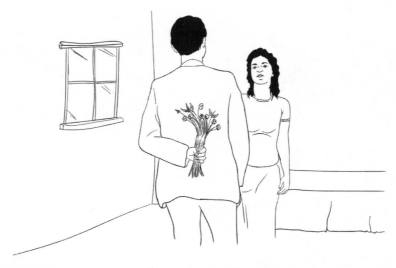

What is this? The technical term for this phenomenon is *hypoactive libido of pregnancy*.

Why is this happening? Hypoactive libido during pregnancy can occur for a variety of reasons, including:

1. Morning sickness: When you feel like crap all day (and frequently all night), the rocking back and forth of sex is the last thing on your mind.

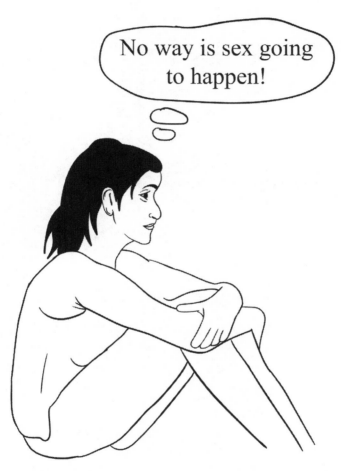

2. Hormonal fluctuations: While for many women these fluctuations cause an increase in libido, for others, it can actually cause your libido to pack its bags and hit the road.

3. Depression: See the section on depression in chapter 18. A common symptom of depression is a decrease in libido and other sexual dysfunctions.

4. Fear of hurting the baby or somehow harming the pregnancy: This is a common but generally unfounded concern unless your provider has instructed otherwise (see the above section Sex During Pregnancy).

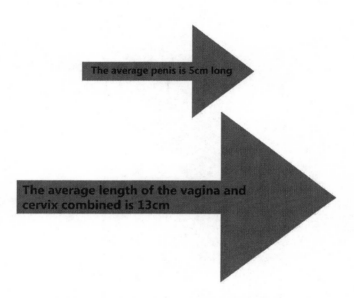

Remember this graphic? The penis can never reach the baby.

Tell me more: Regardless of why your libido has decreased, this lack of desire and intimacy can be a strain on even the strongest relationships, especially if the decrease is not mutual. The good news is that for most people, libido does improve as the pregnancy progresses.

Can I treat this? How you address a decrease in libido really depends upon what's causing it in the first place.

1. **Decreased libido related to depression** needs to be addressed as part of treating the depression, which of course is critically important (see the section on Depression in Pregnancy).

2. **Decreased libido related to hormonal fluctuations** (the most common cause) will usually improve as the second trimester progresses, and the fluctuations start to minimize.

3. **Morning sickness related hypoactive libido** tends to wane as the morning sickness wanes, which for many women is by the end of the first trimester. Not only does your libido tend to return at this point, but there will likely be a significant resurgence in libido as you make up for the lost time.

4. **Fear of hurting the baby:** Hopefully, you have read the Sex During Pregnancy portion of this chapter, if you have, you know that sex will not harm the baby. Even knowing this, for some people, the idea of having sex during pregnancy is a difficult hurdle to overcome. Know that in the absence of high-risk conditions, sex during pregnancy is completely okay and actually beneficial, but at the end of the day, do what makes you and your partner feel most comfortable.

Will this get better? Yes, pregnancy-related hypoactive libido usually improves after delivery. Unfortunately, many people do experience a decrease in libido after delivery as well (sleeplessness, post-delivery discomfort, body image concerns), but that too shall pass. There are some things that you can do in the meantime, however, including:

TO DO LIST

Tip for Daily Living: Make time for "us". Set 30 minutes aside every day just to sit and talk or schedule a date night once per week.

1. **Pregnancy lingerie:** Some women love the way their bodies change during pregnancy; others do not. For some mommies-to-be, pregnancy lingerie bolsters confidence in their sexy new curves.

2. **Time alone:** For many couples, pregnancy is a fun but busy time. A little alone time to reconnect and be physically and emotionally intimate is crucial even if sex doesn't occur.

3. **Just cuddle:** It's okay to cuddle, even if sex doesn't occur. The closeness is physically and emotionally reassuring and comforting to both partners.

When should I call my provider? Anytime you have a concern or question about something, you should discuss it with your provider. If you feel that your decreased libido may be a symptom of depression, or if it is negatively impacting your relationship or sense of wellbeing, contact your provider ASAP.

CHAPTER 18

PREGNANCY AND EMOTIONS

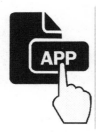 **Don't forget to download the Everything Pregnancy app!**

1). Everyone says I should feel happy, but I just feel sad all of the time.

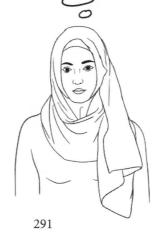

I know this should be one of the happiest times of my life but I am still so sad

Pregnancy and Depression:

Is this real, or am I imagining this? Depression during and after pregnancy is very real. Studies show that up to one-third of all women will experience depression or anxiety during pregnancy.

What is this? The technical name for depression during pregnancy is *peripartum depression,* while depression after delivery is known as *postpartum depression*. Depression is a clinical diagnosis characterized by feelings of sadness, guilt, and hopelessness. We all experience some of these feelings at various points in our life, but the diagnosis of depression is made when feelings are persistent over months, or even years. Symptoms of depression include:

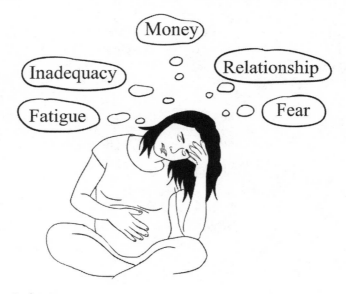

1. Sadness.
2. Hopelessness.
3. Frequent crying.
4. Feelings of guilt.
5. Excessive sleeping, known as *hypersomnia.*
6. Difficulty sleeping, known as *insomnia.*
7. Increased or decreased appetite.

8. Inability to concentrate.

9. Not finding joy in activities that used to be joyful.

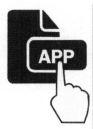

Depression Screen: Be sure to use the Edinburgh Depression Scale section of the app on a regular basis to screen for signs of depression.

TO DO LIST

The time to identify depression is early, when the symptoms may be so subtle that they are missed. Please do the depression screen regularly and share the results with your medical provider.

Why is this happening? *Peripartum and postpartum depression* occur for a multitude of reasons. Frequently a combination of situational factors (fear about the future, feeling overwhelmed, relationship issues, money problems, etc.), and hormonal changes lead to depression. Hormones fluctuate significantly during and after pregnancy, affecting the chemicals in your brain that control your mood.

Tell me more: *Peripartum and postpartum depression* can happen to anyone, but people who have had a history of depression (during a prior pregnancy, after delivery, or completely unrelated to pregnancy) have a higher risk for pregnancy-related depression. *Peripartum depression* can occur at any point during the pregnancy, but the likelihood increases as the pregnancy progresses, and the highest likelihood is actually after delivery.

Old Wives Tale

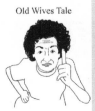

"Depression is a normal part of pregnancy": Depression is not a normal part of pregnancy, and it is not something that you just have to deal with. If you are concerned that you may be suffering from depression, notify your provider immediately!

Can I treat this? Yes, yes, yes. All forms of depression (peripartum, postpartum, and non-pregnancy related) can and absolutely should be treated! Depression is not something that you can just "snap out of." It is an actual medical diagnosis that left untreated can be harmful to mother and baby. Some studies have shown that babies born to mothers with untreated depression have a higher likelihood of premature birth, low birth weight, and increased agitation and irritability. The cornerstones of treating depression are:

1. **Psychotherapy:** Talking to a professional.

2. **Medications called anti-depressants***: Antidepressants help to normalize the levels of certain chemicals in the brain. Thankfully, many antidepressants can be used during pregnancy and while breastfeeding, though as with any medication, you have to discuss risks and benefits with your provider. Antidepressants currently considered safe during pregnancy include:

   ◆ SSRIs (Selective serotonin reuptake inhibitors) like Prozac and Zoloft.

   ◆ SNRIs (Selective norepinephrine reuptake inhibitors) like Cymbalta and Effexor.

   ◆ TCAs (Tricyclic antidepressants) like Amitriptyline.

   ◆ Bupropion.

Old Wives Tale

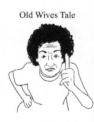

"All anti-depressants are unsafe during pregnancy": Despite what some may believe, many antidepressants can be taken safely during pregnancy and while breastfeeding.

3. **Other alternative options** to treat depression include:

   ◆ Light therapy: Exposure to light, especially in the darker winter months, has been shown to reduce depression.

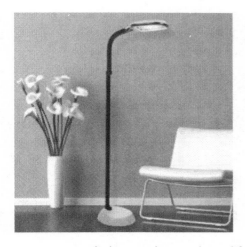 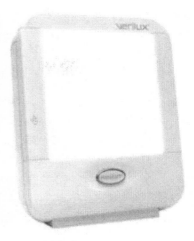

Happy lights can be purchased from many online retailers.

♦ Exercise: The endorphins released during exercise improve mood.

♦ Acupuncture: Acupuncture has been proven in studies to reduce symptoms of depression.

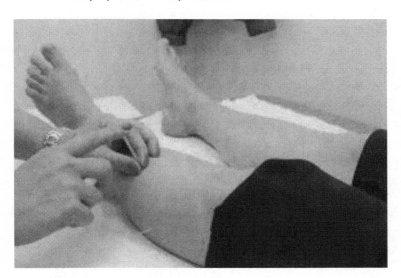

♦ A diet enriched with omega-3 fatty acids.

♦ Getting adequate rest and sleep: Rest, or lack thereof, has also been found to have an effect on the symptoms of depression.

Will this get better? Depression rarely gets better on its own. With proper medical intervention, however, the symptoms of depression can be significantly reduced if not completely eradicated.

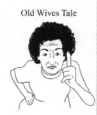

Old Wives Tale

"Depression isn't a real illness, you can just snap out of it if you try!": Depression is not something that you can or will just snap out of and it is not something to be ashamed of. If you are experiencing symptoms of depression, let your medical provider know ASAP!

When should I call my provider? You should call your provider if you experience any of the following:

1. Concern that you might be experiencing depression or symptoms of depression.

2. Thoughts of suicide, homicide, or hearing voices/seeing things that are not there; In these cases, you should inform your provider, and seek emergency care immediately.

2). Why do I always feel so unsettled?

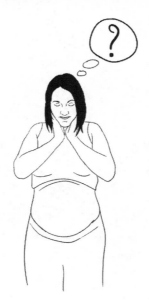

Anxiety and Pregnancy:

296

Is this real, or am I imagining this? Much like depression, anxiety during pregnancy is also a very real thing. Remember, we said that up to one-third of women suffer from depression, or anxiety, or both during pregnancy.

What is this? We all feel anxious from time to time, and pregnancy is rightfully one of these times that will naturally stimulate some anxieties. Will I be a good mom? Can we afford this baby? What will labor be like? Abnormal anxiety, and in particular *generalized anxiety disorder (GAD)*, however, goes above and beyond normal feelings of momentary anxiety. These feelings are intrusive, constant, and difficult to control. All of this makes it very difficult to get through the day normally. Symptoms of generalized anxiety include:

1. Restlessness.
2. Irritability.
3. Feeling overwhelmed.
4. Sleeplessness.
5. Fatigue.
6. Poor concentration.
7. Feeling unable to control worries or fears.
8. Physical symptoms like heart palpitations, a racing heart, muscle tension/ache, and cramping, frequently with diarrhea.

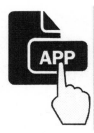

Anxiety Screen: Be sure to complete the anxiety screen on the app.

TO DO LIST

Much like depression, the time to identify and treat anxiety is early. At least once every trimester and again after delivery, take the anxiety screening test in the app and be sure to share the results with your provider.

Why is this happening? Much like Depression, anxiety is in large part related to a combination of life circumstances and the fluctuating hormone levels during and immediately after pregnancy. People who have suffered from generalized anxiety or depression in the past are more likely to be affected, but many women will experience their first symptoms during pregnancy.

Tell me more: The risks of untreated anxiety can actually extend to the developing fetus. Mothers with untreated anxiety have a higher rate of preeclampsia (high blood pressure during pregnancy), which can have adverse effects on mom and baby. Additionally, babies born to mothers with untreated anxiety are more likely to be born prematurely and to have a low birth weight.

Can I treat this? Generalized anxiety can be treated effectively with a combination of psychotherapy (talking to a professional) and medications. Many of the medications used to treat depression can also be used to treat anxiety. Much like depression treatment, you should discuss with your provider about risks and benefits before starting an anti-anxiety treatment regimen. Beyond medications, other options to treat anxiety include:

1. **Exercise:** Increased physical activity during pregnancy is great for overall physical and emotional well-being, and it has been found to reduce the incidence of anxiety.

2. **Sleep:** Get adequate rest, at least 8 hours a night.

3. **Eat a diet with less processed foods:** Studies have found that reducing processed foods can reduce anxiety.

4. **Meditation:** Meditation is good for both short-term and long-term anxiety reduction.

5. **Acupuncture:** Much like depression, acupuncture has also been proven to reduce symptoms of anxiety.

6. **Psychotherapy:** Talk therapy is a great way to get to the root of anxieties.

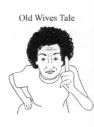

Old Wives Tale

"You are not a mother if you are not always worried": It is not normal to constantly feel anxious or worried. While occasional anxieties are normal in daily life especially concerning pregnancy and delivery, it is not normal to constantly feel anxious or worried. If you do, you should let your provider know immediately.

Will it get better? Without proper acknowledgment and treatment, generalized anxiety frequently does not improve, and it can be harmful to both mother and baby. Addressed and treated appropriately, however, anxiety symptoms much like depression symptoms can be significantly reduced or even eradicated.

When should I call my provider? If you are experiencing any of the symptoms of anxiety mentioned above, especially if they are interfering with your ability to get through your day normally, you should speak with your provider immediately.

3). Clearly there is something wrong with me if I don't already feel a bond with my baby!

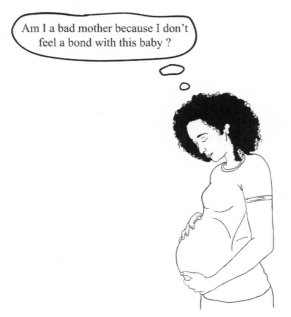

Pregnancy and Bonding.

Is this real, or am I imagining this? No, you are not imagining this. Every pregnancy is different, and every mother-to-be is different, but many pregnant women report having concerns at some time during their pregnancy about not bonding with their babies.

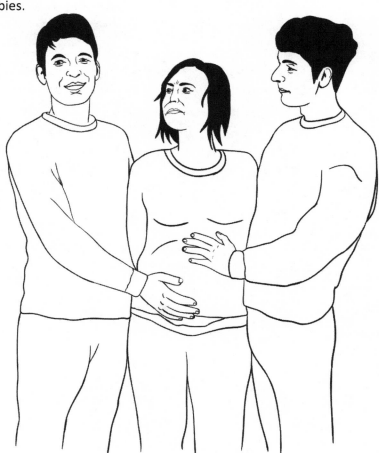

What is this? While no recognized condition interferes with mom's ability to bond with their babies during pregnancy, this situation is more common than you would think (and more common than people like to admit). While most mommies-to-be do experience this at some point, be aware that it can also be a sign of depression (see the section above on Depression).

Why is this happening? There is no single reason why some women don't feel a bond with their baby during pregnancy. Many women, especially first-time moms, report that they have a hard time connecting with an idea that seems so intangible and unreal to them. Others say that they start to feel a connection once they know the baby's gender, while others begin to feel an attachment after the baby has a name. In some of the more extreme instances, women report never feeling bonded with their baby during the pregnancy, stating that they only feel a bond once they actually see and hold their baby.

Tell me more: A lack of bonding with your baby during pregnancy is very common, so don't feel bad. It can, however, be a sign of depression, so be keenly aware, and monitor your symptoms using the Edinburgh Depression scale in the app (see above).

Can I treat this? There are definitely things that you can do to forge that bond with your baby long before he or she makes their entrance into the world, including:

1. **Journaling:** Write a pregnancy journal for your baby, telling her or him about your experiences, thoughts, fears, etc.

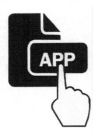

Pregnancy Journal: As hard as this may be to believe, you will actually forget a lot of what you are experiencing now. Journaling is a great way to bond with your growing bundle of joy while preserving this once in a lifetime experience in writing and pictures.

2. **Ultrasound pictures:** Get to know what your baby looks like by frequently looking at ultrasound images, especially pictures of the face.

3. **Talk to your baby:** Your baby is a captive audience, to say the least. Tell him or her all about your day.

4. **Push back:** When your baby communicates with a kick or push, gently respond with a little nudge. This is a special connection that only the two of you share.

5. **Give your baby a name or a nickname:** Naming your baby makes her or him feel more real. Give the baby a name even if you change your mind later.

6. **Find out the gender:** Knowing if you are having a daughter or a son makes the idea of her or him more tangible.

7. **Play music for your baby:** Enjoy nice, soothing music with your baby. Both of you will appreciate it, and it is a nice, quiet time just to get to know one another.

TO DO LIST

Studies have shown that children whose parents exposed them to music in utero, especially classical music, have higher IQs, so listen to music at least 30 minutes every day.

8. **Daydream:** Introduce yourself to your baby in your head, and get to know her or him by daydreaming about what life will be like with them.

Will it get better? Rest assured that the bonding will come. They call mothers "mama bears" for a reason, and it has very little to do with hibernation!

When should I call my provider? If you are concerned about your lack of bonding with your baby (before or after delivery), or if you experience symptoms of depression and/or anxiety related to this or other issues, contact your provider.

CHAPTER 19

EXERCISE, WEIGHT, AND PREGNANCY

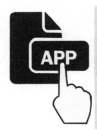

Don't forget to download the Everything Pregnancy app!

1). How much weight should I gain during pregnancy?

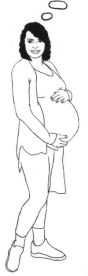

Normal Weight Gain During Pregnancy:

Is this real, or am I imagining this? Many pregnant women are concerned that they might be gaining too much weight when, in fact, their weight gain is completely normal. This is usually compounded by the fact that people often comment about the size of a pregnant woman's belly. By now you've probably heard a comment like "It looks like you are going to pop any day now!" Or, "Are you sure you're not having twins?" So no, you are not imagining this, it is completely normal to be concerned about your weight gain.

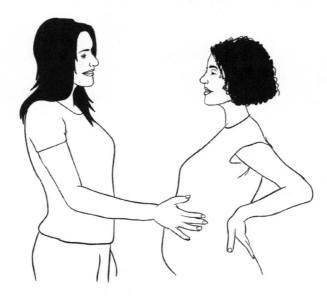

Why is this happening? Gaining weight during pregnancy is normal; after all, you are carrying another growing human being in your body. Every woman's weight gain is different, but in general, you should gain between 15-40 pounds over the entire pregnancy. Your expected weight gain is determined primarily by your starting weight and specifically your BMI (Body Mass Index).

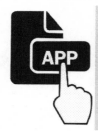

Use the app's BMI (body mass index) calculator to determine what your current BMI is and what your ideal BMI range is.

Tell me more: These are guidelines for weight gain but remember every woman and every pregnancy is different, so don't freak out if your weight gain numbers and pattern are a little different.

1. **If your BMI before pregnancy was within the normal range (18.5-24.9),** you should gain between 25-35 pounds during the entire pregnancy. For twin pregnancies, you should gain between 37-54 pounds over the entire pregnancy.

   ◆ First trimester (0-13 6/7 weeks): 2-3 pounds total.

   ◆ Second (14-27 6/7 weeks) and third (28 weeks to birth) trimesters: 1 pound per week.

2. **If your BMI was in the underweight range before pregnancy (less than 18.5),** you should gain 28-40 pounds during the entire pregnancy. For twin pregnancies, you should gain 50-62 pounds during the entire pregnancy.
   ◆ First trimester: 3-4 pounds in total.
   ◆ Second and third trimesters: 1 pound per week.

3. **If your BMI was in the overweight range before pregnancy (25-29.9)**, you should gain 15-25 pounds over the entire pregnancy. For twin pregnancies, you should gain between 31-50
   ◆ First trimester: 1-2 pounds total.
   ◆ Second and third trimesters: ½ pound per week.

4. **If your BMI was in the obese range before pregnancy (30 or more),** you should gain 10-20 pounds during the entire pregnancy. For twin pregnancies, you should gain between 25-42 pounds over the entire pregnancy.

   ◆ First trimester: Approximately 1 pound total.

   ◆ Second and third trimesters: ½ pound per week.

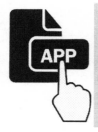

Use the app's Weight Tracker to record your starting weight and monitor your weight gain during your pregnancy.

Old Wives Tale

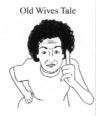

"Don't count your calories, just eat!": Sorry, pregnancy does not give you carte blanche to eat whatever you want, whenever you want. Keep your diet clean and healthy with just one or two splurge days per week.

Can I treat this? Well, if your weight gain is normal, there is nothing to treat, so just sit back, relax, and enjoy this extraordinary experience. If your weight gain is abnormal (too much or too little) check out the sections that follow.

Will this get better? Again, if your weight gain is normal, there is nothing to worry about. See the sections that follow if your weight gain is excessive or insufficient.

When should I call my provider? Always communicate with your provider if you have any questions or concerns. If you feel like your weight gain is too much or too little (see the sections that follow), you should definitely speak with your provider.

2). Why should I gain 35 pounds when the baby only weighs 7 pounds?!

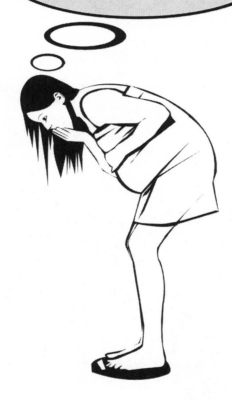

Where Does All of This Pregnancy Weight Gain Go Anyway?

Is this real, or am I imagining this? This is absolutely a valid question; how can it be "normal" to gain up to 40 pounds when the average baby only weighs about 7 pounds?

Why is this happening? While the baby accounts for a portion of the weight you will gain during pregnancy; there are a lot of other things happening in your body that account for the additional weight.

Tell me more: Well, there is a lot more to pregnancy than just that cute little baby that you are growing, and these things account for the additional weight gained. The body has to make a lot of changes to make sure that your bundle of joy is healthy, both during and after pregnancy. Again, every woman and every pregnancy is different, but this is a rough breakdown of where that extra non-baby weight is coming from:

1. Uterus— 2-3 pounds: After all, the uterus goes from the size of a walnut before pregnancy to the size of a watermelon at the time of delivery.

2. Increased blood volume, 3 pounds: Your blood volume increases so that your body can effectively support your needs as well as the needs of your baby.

3. Breasts— 1 pound: Breast enlargement occurs as your body prepares for lactation.

4. Placenta— 2-3 pounds.

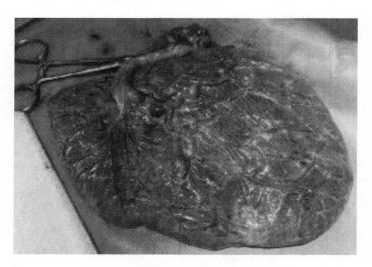

A full-term placenta.

5. Amniotic fluid— 2-3 pounds.

6. Extra fat tissue— 5 pounds: Fear not though; this excess fatty tissue is a much-needed source of energy for both mom and baby.

7. Fluid retention— 5 pounds: Sorry to break it to you, but retaining fluid, especially in the lower extremities, is a normal part of pregnancy.

TO DO LIST

Tips for Daily Living: If you notice some swelling of the lower extremities you can:

#1. Wear support hose.

#2. Wear a belly belt.

#3. Reduce salt intake.

#4. Elevate your legs whenever able.

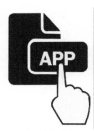

Don't forget to check out the BMI calculator and Weight Tracker features of the app!

Can I treat this? You already know the answer to this question; if your weight gain is within the normal range, there is nothing to treat.

Will this get better? Again, if your weight gain is within the normal range, there is nothing to worry about and nothing that needs to get better. Generally, weight gain that is within the desired range will completely resolve by 6-12 weeks postpartum, especially if you breastfeed and remain active after delivery.

When should I call my provider? If you have abnormal (too much or too little) weight gain, communicate with your provider, especially if you notice a sudden onset of weight gain or fluid retention.

3). Yayyy, pregnancy, now I can eat whatever I want, whenever I want!

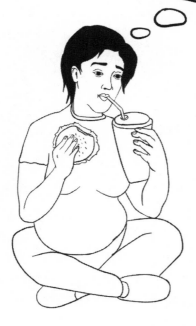

Woohoo, I'm pregnant now so that means that I can have a cheeseburger and a milkshake for breakfast, right?

Pregnancy and Over-Eating?

Is this real, or am I imagining this? Many mommies-to-be think that being pregnant means they can eat whatever they want whenever they want. So, if this is you, you are not imagining this, but you are mistaken!

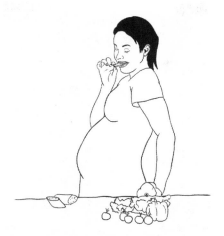

Why is this happening? Some women take the term "eating for two" seriously, and they really believe they need to eat for two. I hate to be the buster of bubbles, but during pregnancy, your body only requires an additional 300 calories per day to support its changing needs. For twin pregnancies, that number is closer to an extra 500 calories per day. During the third trimester, this number is a little bit higher at 400 calories per day for single pregnancies and 600 calories per day for twin pregnancies.

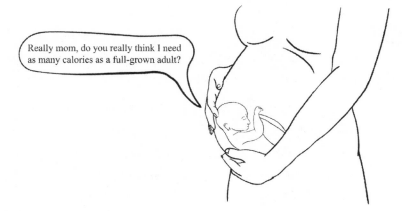

Really mom, do you really think I need as many calories as a full-grown adult?

Tell me more: You have to know how many calories you should be eating daily before pregnancy to know how many calories you should be eating during pregnancy. Again, every woman is different, but a moderately active woman will need about 2,200 calories per day before pregnancy while a more sedentary woman, will only need about 2,000 calories per day. Total calories are important, but

311

you should also know the 20/30/50 rule. Roughly 20% of your calories should come from proteins, 30% from fats, and 50% from carbohydrates.

I know, we are so mean teasing you with a pie chart that is an actual pie chart. Bet you want some pie now, don't you?

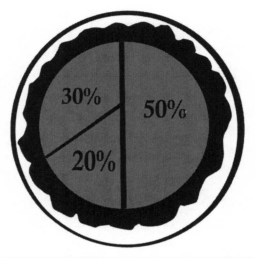

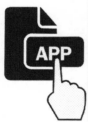
Be sure to use the Food and Fitness Tracker every day. It will keep you honest and on track with your eating habits.

Can I treat this? Yep, just monitor how many calories you are eating per day, and make sure that you are distributing them accordingly between calories from proteins, fats, and carbs.

Old Wives Tale

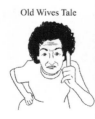
"You can eat whatever you want during pregnancy!" Sorry, but we have to restate it, that old wife is a liar, and you cannot eat whatever you want whenever you want!

Will this get better? Let's be honest folks, it doesn't matter if you are female or male, pregnant or not pregnant, we all like to eat, and we all look for excuses to overeat. So no, that desire to overeat will likely not get better; eating well is a daily struggle.

When should I call my provider? If you have questions or concerns about proper nutrition during pregnancy, you should contact your provider.

4). How did I gain 6 pounds in one week?!

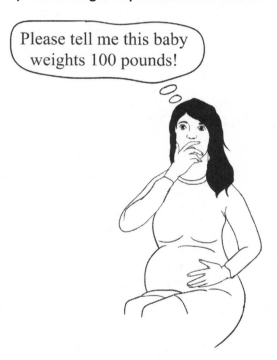

Excessive Weight Gain During Pregnancy:

TO DO LIST

Tip for daily living: Go for stronger flavors and try adding a touch of ginger.

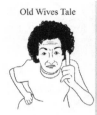

"Don't worry about how much weight you are gaining": DO NOT listen to this old wife; it is not okay to eat whatever, and whenever, you want to during pregnancy! Newsflash, you are NOT really eating for two.

Is this real, or am I imagining this? While we can guarantee you that your baby will be tons of fun, he or she won't literally be *tons* of fun, so if your weight gain has gone beyond the parameters discussed earlier, then you are not imagining this, and the excessive weight gain is real.

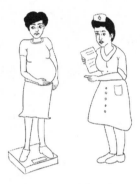

Why is it happening? There are many reasons for excessive weight gain during pregnancy, but the single biggest reason is over-eating (we're sorry to have to break it to you). As we previously discussed, most mommies-to-be only need an additional 300-400 calories per day, depending upon the trimester of pregnancy and how many babies you are carrying. Anything beyond this is over-eating.

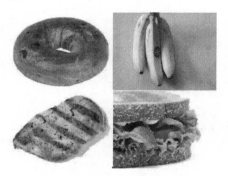

Foods that each represent 300-400 calories (a bagel, three bananas, a turkey sandwich, two breasts of chicken)

314

Tell me more: Excessive weight gain during pregnancy is a concern for both mom and baby. Babies born to mothers who've gained too much weight have a higher risk of also being overweight at birth, which means a higher rate of C-section and/or maternal pelvic damage. Babies born to mothers who've gained too much weight during pregnancy also have higher rates of lifelong obesity and diabetes.

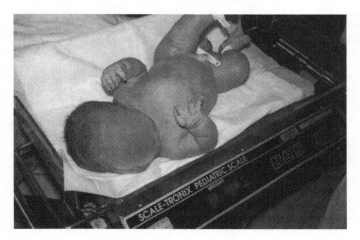

This macrosomic (large) baby weighed 11 pounds at birth.

Beyond excessive caloric intake, other potential causes of excessive weight gain during pregnancy include preeclampsia, gestational diabetes, and polyhydramnios.

1. Preeclampsia: Preeclampsia is a condition characterized by high blood pressure, amongst other things, during pregnancy. Preeclampsia tends to occur during the third trimester, and it causes excessive weight gain due primarily to fluid retention. For more details, refer to the section on preeclampsia.

2. Gestational diabetes/Polyhydramnios: This is a less common cause of excessive weight gain. Gestational diabetes is diabetes specific to pregnancy, and polyhydramnios is over-production of amniotic fluid, which can occur when blood sugar is higher than it should be.

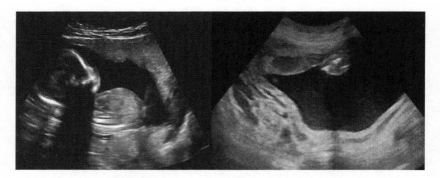

Notice the difference between normal amniotic fluid (the black liquid) on the left and excessive amniotic fluid on the right.

Can I treat this? The ability to treat excessive weight gain depends upon the cause. Medical conditions like preeclampsia and gestational diabetes require medical intervention (again, refer to the sections for these specific conditions). When it comes to the most common cause, over-eating, here are a few tips that can help to curb your weight gain:

1. **Eat smaller meals more frequently:** Instead of having three large meals, have 5-6 smaller meals throughout the day, making sure that your total caloric intake does not exceed the recommendations that we discussed earlier in this chapter.

2. **Hydrate, hydrate, hydrate:** Hydration is super important during pregnancy for a variety of reasons, including reduction of bladder/kidney infections and reduction of preterm labor risk. Adequate hydration also reduces hunger, which helps with maintaining a healthy weight.

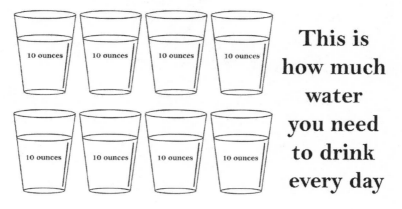

This is how much water you need to drink every day

3. **Cut the empty calories:** Replace food like French fries, potato chips, and cookies with fruits, vegetables, and whole grains.

4. **Make sure that you are eating foods high in protein and healthy fats:** Proteins are good for you and your growing baby, and they also help to curb the appetite. Healthy fats include polyunsaturated fats, nuts, seeds, and vegetable oils.

5. **Get active and stay active:** Pregnancy is not the time to become sedentary. Daily (preferably) or near daily, moderate exercise during pregnancy helps to maintain a healthy weight while also reducing the risk of high blood pressure and diabetes. As a nice cherry on top, physical activity during pregnancy has been linked to faster labors.

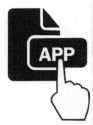

Be sure to use the Food and Fitness Tracker every day. It will keep you honest and on track with your eating habits.

Will this get better? This is one of those rare times when we have to say that in the absence of intervention, this problem likely will not improve. Excessive weight gain related to medical conditions like preeclampsia and gestational diabetes/polyhydramnios improve after delivery, but excessive weight gain caused by over-eating not only doesn't improve after delivery, but many studies show that it usually worsens, increasing the likelihood of life-long obesity and obesity-related conditions like type 2 diabetes and hypertension.

When should I call my provider? Any time you have excessive weight gain, you should discuss that with your provider. If the excessive weight gain is sudden or associated with excessive fluid retention, especially in the last trimester of pregnancy, you should contact your provider immediately as these can be signs of Preeclampsia.

5). I thought I would have gained more weight by now.

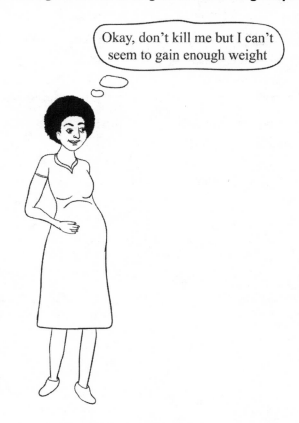

Inadequate Weight Gain During Pregnancy:

Is this real, or am I imagining this? Believe it or not, the problem of not gaining enough weight during pregnancy is not as uncommon as some might think. If you are gaining less weight than the recommendations previously discussed, you likely have inadequate pregnancy weight gain.

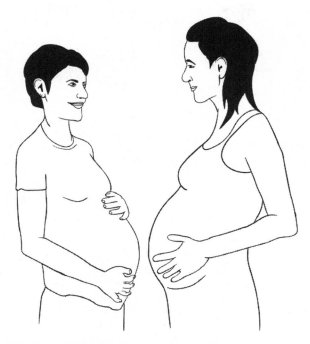

Why is this happening? Don't fret if you are not gaining weight or even if you are losing weight during the first trimester. Lack of weight gain or some weight loss during the first trimester is common and is usually due to the nausea and vomiting that most pregnant women experience during early pregnancy. Beyond the first trimester, however, inadequate weight gain is a serious concern and is usually due to either poor nutrition or taking in an insufficient number of daily calories. Beyond nutritional issues, poor weight gain can be a symptom of certain medical conditions like hyperthyroidism (an overactive thyroid) as well as anxiety or depression, though these tend to be exceptions to the rule.

Tell me more: Poor weight gain beyond the first trimester is a huge concern because babies born to mothers who gained less than the recommended amount of weight have a higher risk of IUGR (intrauterine growth restriction), which results in smaller than average babies; and they have a higher risk of IUFD (intrauterine fetal demise), which is the death of a baby before birth.

Can I treat this? This can be treated, but the *how* is determined by the *why*:

1. **In the vast majority of cases, the treatment for poor weight gain is merely increasing caloric intake.** You just want to make sure that those new calories come from healthy, nutritious food sources, and no, pizza and milkshakes, despite their dairy content, don't count!

    ♦ *A moderately active woman (most women)* should be eating approximately 2500 calories per day during the first and second trimesters of pregnancy and 2600 calories per day during the last trimester of pregnancy. Women who are overweight/obese or underweight before pregnancy will need to eat fewer or more calories, respectively. In these cases, it is important that you discuss your specific recommendations with your provider.

    ♦ *A more sedentary woman* should be eating 2300 calories per day during the first and second trimesters of pregnancy and 2400 calories per day during the last trimester of pregnancy. Again, women who are overweight/obese or underweight before pregnancy will need to eat fewer or more calories, respectively. In these cases, it is important that you discuss your specific recommendations with your provider.

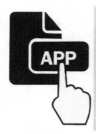

Be sure to use the Food and Fitness Tracker every day. It will keep you honest and on track with your eating habits and monitoring your weight gain.

2. **Other less common causes of poor weight gain like hyperthyroidism, anxiety, or depression require medical treatment.** Hyperthyroidism is usually treated with medications to reduce the activity of your thyroid gland, while anxiety and depression are typically treated with a combination of medication and talk therapy.

Will this get better? With appropriate management, poor weight gain should improve.

When should I call my Provider? Your provider should be monitoring your weight closely throughout your pregnancy, but any time you have a concern, you should communicate that with your provider.

6). Do I have to stop exercising now that I am pregnant?

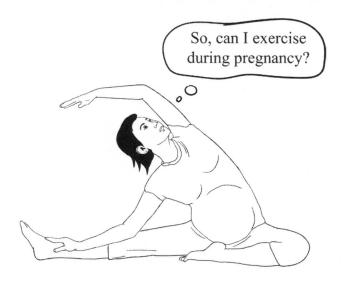

Exercise and Pregnancy:

Not only *can* you exercise during pregnancy (with very few exceptions), you actually *should* exercise during pregnancy. We all know that regular exercise is generally seen as a good thing. Well, guess what? The benefits of regular exercise only increase during pregnancy. Now, before you start, continue, or change your pre-pregnancy exercise routine, it is important that you discuss the specifics with your provider first.

Old Wives Tale

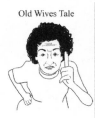

"Pregnancy means always staying off of your feet": Pregnancy is not the time to relax and kick your feet up! Pregnancy is a well state and you should stay active all pregnancy long!

7). What are the rules of exercise during pregnancy?

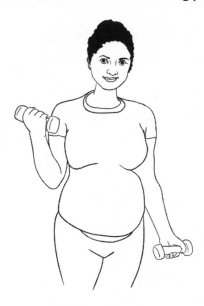

Keeping Exercise Safe During Pregnancy:

As a general rule, any exercise that does not pose a risk of trauma or injury to your growing baby bump is safe during pregnancy. Having said that, there are some other important things to keep in mind.

1. **If you were physically active before pregnancy,** you generally do not want to increase your level of activity during pregnancy significantly. In other words, keep it steady, and wait until after delivery to push yourself harder. If you were doing an hour in the gym before pregnancy, don't do more than an hour in the gym during pregnancy.

2. **If you were not physically active before pregnancy,** start with a low to moderate level of exercise. As a general rule of thumb, 30 minutes per day of activities that get your heart rate up and cause you to break a sweat while still being able to talk would be a good starting point.

3. **Hydration** is always crucial during pregnancy, and this is especially the case before and during exercise.

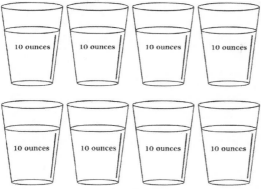

This is how much water you need to drink every day

4. **Keep your heart rate at or below 150.**

5. **Don't do exercises that carry a potential risk of abdominal trauma (i.e., sit-ups, pushups, etc.).**

6. **Don't do exercises where balance is integral** (i.e., roller skating and non-stationary bike riding) because your balance will definitely be taking a vacation as your pregnancy progresses.

7. **Avoid contact sports.**

8. **Avoid heights and depths,** so no sky-diving and no scuba diving. The pressure changes aren't good for your bundle of joy.

9. **Keep it cool.** No hot yoga or hot Pilates.

TO DO LIST

Tips for Daily Living:

#1. Exercise at least 30 minutes on most days with your medical providers okay.

#2. Stay well hydrated at all times, especially when you exercise.

#3. Keep it cool and on two feet.

#4. Elevate your legs whenever able.

8). Why should I exercise during pregnancy?

The Benefits of Exercise During Pregnancy:

Exercise during pregnancy has tons of physical and emotional benefits, some of which you probably never knew, including:

1. Improved mood and sense of wellbeing.

2. Less depression during pregnancy and postpartum.

3. Keeping weight gain during pregnancy under control.

4. Faster and more significant weight loss after delivery.

5. Reduced incidence of gestational diabetes.

6. Reduced incidence of hypertension and Preeclampsia.

7. Shorter labors.

8. Quicker deliveries with less need for interventions like forceps or vacuum deliveries as well as fewer cesarean sections.

9. Reduced post-partum pain and discomfort.

9). When should I slow things down in the gym?

Warning Signs to Look for While Exercising During Pregnancy:

If you experience any of the following during exercise, stop and immediately contact your provider:

1. Vaginal bleeding or leakage of fluid from the vagina.

2. Regular contractions, persistent cramping, or persistent abdominal or back pain.

3. Dizziness.

4. Headaches.

5. Chest pain.

6. Extreme leg pain and/or swelling.

10). When is it okay not to exercise?

You May Be Excused:

While we advocate exercise for most pregnant women, there are times when exercise should be modified or avoided altogether during pregnancy. If you have any of the following conditions, you will want to speak to your provider before exercising:

1. Hypertension and/or preeclampsia.

2. Preterm labor.

3. Rupture of membranes (broken bag of water).

4. Placental issues, including previa (when the placenta covers the cervix) and abruption (when the placenta starts to detach from the uterine wall prematurely).

5. Severe anemia.

6. Cervical incompetence/insufficiency (when the cervix dilates too early), or if you have a cerclage in place (a stitch to close the cervix).

7. Heart or lung disease.

8. Vaginal bleeding.

PLACENTA PREVIA

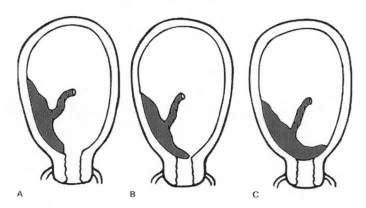

A-Low lying placenta (close to the cervix), B-Marginal previa (partially covering the cervix), C-Complete previa (completely covering the cervix).

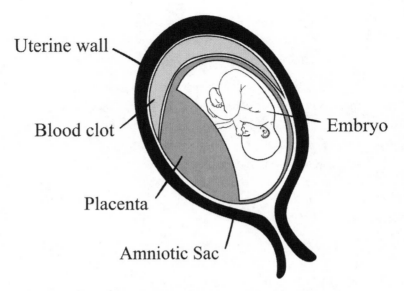

Uterine wall

Blood clot

Placenta

Amniotic Sac

Embryo

Placental abruption occurs when the placenta separates from the uterine wall too early.

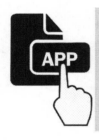

APP

Be sure to use the Fitness Tracker feature of the app to track your food and calories as well as your daily exercise and activity.

CHAPTER 20

GETTING READY FOR THE BIG DAY

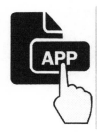

Don't forget to download the Everything Pregnancy app!

1). What is a birth plan, and do I really need one?

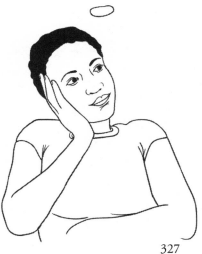

Should I create a birth plan and what is a birth plan anyway?

The Birth Plan:

We bet this journey has seemed more like a slow, lumbering trot than a marathon, but believe it or not, it is quickly coming to an end! If you have dared to take a peek at Chapter 20, this means that you are starting to get ready for the hospital, and it's now time to start thinking about how this is all going to end. So, grab a nice cup of tea, curl up in your favorite chair, and let's get ready for that all-important trip to the hospital or birthing center! It goes without saying that every family's birth experience will be unique to that family, and really that's part of the beauty of the whole process, but a little bit of preparation and pre-planning will help ensure that your birth experience is the best possible experience for your new family.

Let's start at the beginning— what exactly is a birth plan? A birth plan is a written document that discusses exactly how you want your labor and delivery process to go. Depending on your desires, it can be long and detailed, or it can be short and to the point. Whether or not you even have a birthing plan is entirely up to you. Regardless of what you decide, we always stress to mommies-to-be and families-to-be that labor and delivery are always unpredictable, and there are times when the plan may have to change on short notice. Having an idea of what you want, what you don't want, and sharing that with your provider is a key part of empowering yourself and your family to have the labor and delivery experience that you desire. At the same time, having the flexibility and willingness to make changes on short notice is also something you should prepare for.

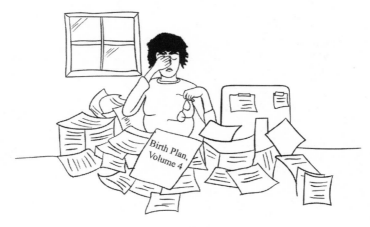

What are some things that might be included in a birth plan? As we said, a birth plan is a very individualized document written by you, the patient, and your support partner, so really, the sky is the limit. Some common things that you might find on a birth plan include:

1. **Pain control:** Is pain medication during labor a must? Do you want to leave your options open when the time actually comes, or do you absolutely want a pain medication-free labor and delivery? If you want pain medications, do you want IV pain medication, or do you want an epidural? If you haven't already, be sure to check out Chapter 22 to learn all about your pain control options during labor.

2. **Ambulation***:* As long as it is safe for you and baby, do you want to be up and moving during labor, or would you prefer to labor in your bed? Ambulation has some definite benefits when it comes to managing pain and speeding labor along, so be sure to read about these in Chapter 22.

3. **Labor-inducing/augmenting medications:** There are times when induction of labor is necessary, but there are also times when it is purely optional. Some mommies-to-be want to have their labor induced, while others want to wait for labor to start on its own. If optional, do you want labor to be induced, or do you want to wait for it to occur on its own? If you opt for labor induction, or if labor has to be induced, do you have a preference when it comes to induction methods? There is a lot that goes into choosing a particular labor induction method, so this is a discussion that you will definitely need to have with your provider. Labor induction methods include:

   ♦ *Nipple stimulation:* This causes the body to produce the hormone *oxytocin*, which can stimulate contractions.

   ♦ *Cytotec:* This is a pill placed in the vagina that contains synthetic prostaglandins, chemicals the body normally produces to prepare the cervix for labor while also stimulating contractions.

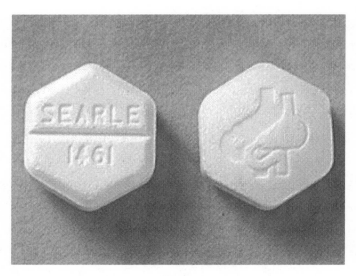

Cytotec.

♦ **Cervidil:** Like Cytotec, Cervidil is a form of synthetic prostaglandin that is placed in the vagina to stimulate contractions and prepare the cervix for labor. Unlike Cytotec, Cervidil is a string, not a pill.

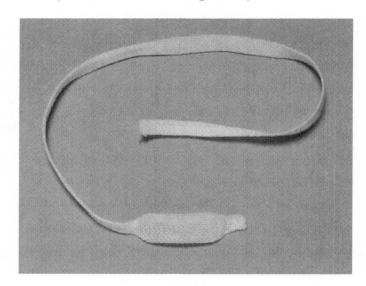

Cervidil.

♦ **Cervical Foley Balloon:** This is a balloon that is placed in the cervix to mechanically dilate it while also causing the body to produce prostaglandins that ready the cervix for labor and stimulate contractions.

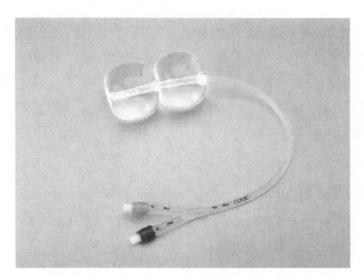

Cervical ripening balloon.

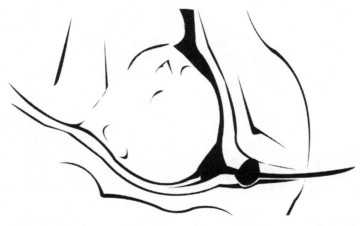

Generally, one balloon is above the cervix and one below, compressing the cervix.

♦ **Pitocin:** Pitocin is an IV medication that is the synthetic form of *oxytocin,* the hormone that the brain secretes to start contractions and labor.

4. **Monitoring (fetal and uterine):** Do you want your baby's heart rate and your contraction pattern monitored continuously or intermittently (usually only an option in lower risk pregnancies)? When it comes to monitoring, are you okay with both internal and external monitors if needed?

    ♦   ***External Monitors:*** These are belts that are placed over the abdomen to monitor and register both the baby's heart rate and the frequency of your contractions.

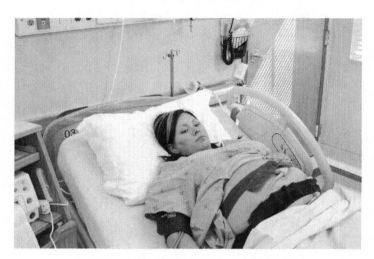

The top belt monitors contractions while the bottom belt monitors your baby's heartbeat.

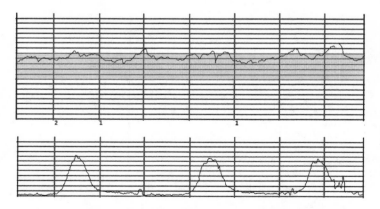

Fetal and uterine tracing: The top line traces the baby's heart rate while the bottom line traces contractions.

- ♦ **Internal Monitors**: Internal monitors are placed directly into the uterus when external monitors are not able to provide the necessary information. These monitors can only be placed once the bag of water is broken, and they provide more accurate measurements of both the baby's heart rate and mom's contractions.

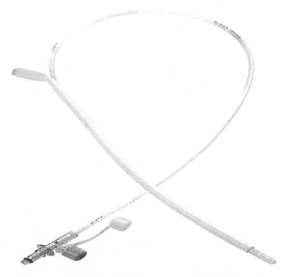

IUPC: Intrauterine pressure catheter that can be placed in the uterus to measure the timing and strength of contractions.

5. **IV access:** Most providers will want an IV placed in case of an emergency even if you don't receive any medications through it.

6. **Food and beverages:** Every provider is different when it comes to their preferences regarding eating and drinking during labor. We tend to recommend that laboring mothers be allowed to eat and drink during early labor and that they restrict themselves to only liquids and very light snacks during active labor. For pregnancies with a higher risk of cesarean section, eating and drinking will likely need to be restricted. We discuss this more in Chapter 22.

7. **Support person:** Who do you want with you during the labor and delivery process? This pertains to not only who is with you in the delivery room, but also who is with you in the operating room if a cesarean delivery becomes necessary.

8. **Birth position:** There are a variety of positions that women like during labor and delivery, including on the back, squatting, or on the hands and knees. These are discussed in greater detail in Chapter 22. If you have a preference, you'll want to include that in your birthing plan.

9. **Cord clamping:** Do you want the umbilical cord clamping to be delayed, or do you want the cord clamped and cut immediately after delivery? Some of the benefits of delayed cord clamping (waiting 3-5 minutes after delivery or until the cord stops pulsing on its own) include increased infant blood volume, decreased infant anemia, and according to some studies, improved long-term neurodevelopment (brain and nerves).

10. **Skin-to-skin contact:** Do you want your baby placed immediately on your chest after delivery, or do you want her or him taken to the warmer first? Many studies suggest that immediate skin-to-skin contact improves bonding between mother and baby, helps baby keep his or her body temperature up, and facilitates easier initiation of breastfeeding.

11. **Immediate or delayed bath:** More and more hospitals are delaying baby's first bath until 24 hours after delivery. Some studies have shown that delaying the first bath for 24-48 hours improves the baby's immune system, improves his or her ability to maintain normal body temperature, and also helps to stabilize baby's blood sugar levels.

12. **Breastfeeding, bottle-feeding or both:** In general, exclusive breastfeeding is the best option for both mommy and baby, but every mother and every baby is different, and the choice is yours. Whatever your choice, discuss it with your provider and make your wishes known.

13. **Circumcision (for male infants):** Do you want your baby circumcised, and if so, do you want the circumcision done while the baby is still in the hospital or later? Some of the benefits of circumcision according to the American Academy of Pediatricians include reduced risk of contracting and transmitting STIs (sexually transmitted infections) later in life, reduced risk of cancer of the penis, and reduced risk of cervical cancer for sexual partners.

14. **Who will stay with the baby after birth:** Many parents want at least one parent to remain with the baby at all times if possible.

15. **Comfort measures (special music, oils, scents, pictures, etc.):** If there is anything that you would like to bring with you for comfort, let your healthcare provider and the labor and delivery team know.

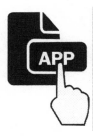

Be sure to use the Birth Plan feature of the app located in the Getting Ready for Delivery section to develop, save and print your birth plan.

TO DO LIST

Before starting your birth plan checkout Chapter 26. Chapter 26 is all about working through and writing your birthing plan.

2). Should I see where I'm going to deliver before I go into labor?

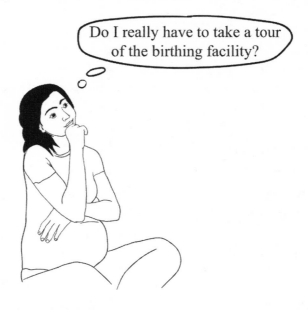

Touring Your Birth Facility:

Labor and Delivery isn't a "medical procedure"; it's a natural process and the birth of a family. A huge part of having a comfortable and memorable experience is feeling comfortable and familiar in your environment. Most labor and delivery facilities (hospital or birthing center) are made to feel warm and cozy, but every facility, like every patient, is different and what feels comfortable to one person may not feel as comfortable to another. Ask to see the labor and delivery suites, the post-partum rooms, the infant nursery, the C-section suite (be prepared for everything), as well as the waiting facilities for family members. Remember, most providers can deliver at multiple locations, so if one place doesn't feel right, tour the other available facilities.

TO DO LIST

It's a good idea to take a tour of the labor and delivery facility early in the third trimester. If it doesn't feel comfortable, inquire about other possible birthing locations.

3). What can I really learn at childbirth education classes?

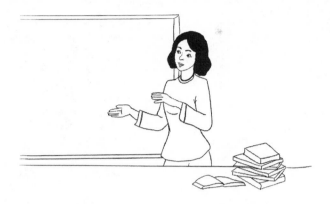

Childbirth Education Classes:

Many expectant parents (especially first-time mommies and daddies) say that taking a birthing education class made them feel more prepared for the whole experience. Childbirth education classes are generally offered weekly for a defined period of time (4-6 weeks) or as a condensed weekend course. Birthing classes will review everything from preparing for labor, breathing techniques, and other pain control methods while in labor to what exactly to expect during delivery and in the hours and days after birth. Birthing classes are an excellent way for the entire birth team (support person and other family members) to become involved and learn things that they can do to make the process smoother and more enjoyable. Most providers or birth facilities will have childbirth education classes, so be sure to ask your provider for specific details.

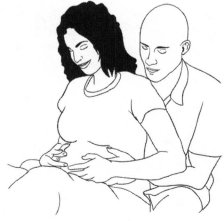

Start looking for childbirth education classes as you near the end of the second trimester, usually between 24 and 28 weeks of pregnancy.

4). Okay, what should go into my labor bag?

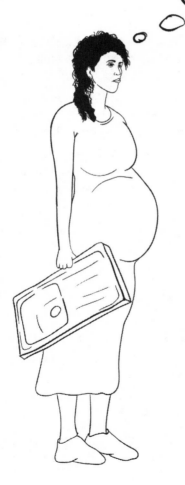

Packing That Labor Bag:

Many parents-to-be spend a lot of time thinking about what to pack in that all-important labor bag. Take it from the TwinDocs, spend less time thinking about the bag and more time enjoying these last few baby-free moments. See a movie, go to dinner, heck even sleep in, or take a nice, long nap. The labor bag is probably one of the most overblown things, and as a rule, simple is always better. Most hospitals and birthing centers do a great job of anticipating and meeting the needs of new families, and to be honest, there just isn't much that you will need to bring along. So, having said all of that, what are some things you should consider packing?

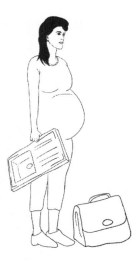

1. **Phone numbers** for your provider as well as the phone number and address for the hospital/birthing center. Hopefully, you already have this information stored on your phone in our handy dandy app, but a written backup is also nice to have.

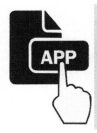

Be sure to record all important phone numbers (loved ones, medical provider, birthing location) in the Important Numbers section of the app.

2. **A copy of your birth plan** if you have one. Again, we hope you have filled this out and stored it in our handy dandy app, but make sure to have a paper copy as well.

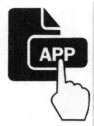

Be sure to use the Birth Plan feature of the app located in the Getting Ready for Delivery section. Here you can develop, save and print your birth plan.

3. **Snacks** for you and your support person. The hospital/birthing center will feed you and will usually provide food for your support person as well, but we can't vouch for the quality; plus, you will likely want a little snack at odd hours. Remember, don't eat if your provider or nurse has told you not to.

4. **CAMERA AND CHARGER!** Yes, we bolded that and added the exclamation mark! This is a once in a lifetime experience (at least for this particular child), and if you don't capture it at the moment, there is no going back!

5. **Chargers** for your phones, laptops, and other electronics.

6. **Good reading material to pass the time** since there will probably be a lot of downtime. A good magazine, book, or even board game can make time fly.

7. **Socks** to keep your tootsies warm and toasty, but only wear your personal socks when you are wearing slippers. Otherwise, just wear the grippy socks that the hospital or birthing center will provide to prevent falls.

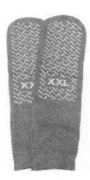

8. **Slippers** just in case you don't want to walk the halls in the provided grippy socks.

9. **A comfy robe** will give you some much-needed coverage since most ladies don't like the butt-out look of traditional medical gowns.

10. **Shower shoes** are always a good idea when you're using a public shower, even if you are not type-A like us. Though you will be the only person using the shower at that time, it is still a public shower, and it's always a good idea to wear shower shoes to prevent possible foot infections.

11. **Your favorite soap, shampoo, and lotion** are essentials to pack if you have allergies or are just particular and don't want to use what the hospital or birthing center will provide.

12. **A change of clothes to go home in**. Sometimes labor can be messy, and you may not want to wear the same clothes home that you wore to the hospital or birthing center. And don't forget to include a clean change of underwear in that bag because your old undies will have been on the front line and may be soiled.

13. **A change of clothes for the support person as well** since labor isn't always just messy for mom. If your support person plans to stay at the hospital or birthing center the entire time after delivery, be sure to bring multiple changes of clothes.

14. **PJs** are a comfort many new moms prefer to the gowns or clothing provided by the hospital or birthing center. Just remember, bleeding after delivery tends to be heavy, so don't bring anything that you absolutely don't want to have to throw away.

15. **Baby's going home outfit** is a must-have. Make it cute because this is what your new bundle of joy will be wearing for her or his debut to the outside world.

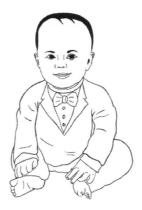

16. **Any comfort items that you may want during labor** should be in your labor bag. This could include candles (check with the hospital or birthing center's policy), music (see if they have a CD or MP3 player, or determine if you need your own), pictures, flowers; you name it. Bring whatever will make your environment feel more comfy and homelike, within reason, of course.

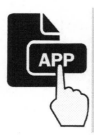

Use the Labor Bag Checklist section of the app to make sure that you don't forget to pack something important!

TO DO LIST

Go ahead and pack that labor bag early in the third trimester (by 32 weeks). Only 10% of babies are actually born on their due date; some come early, and some come late. Packing that bag early will tick one more box off of your list while making sure you are ready if your bundle of joy decides to make an early entrance.

5). What are some common things that people pack that are just unnecessary?

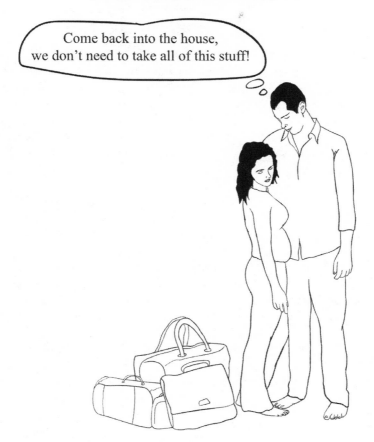

Things That Just Don't Need to Be in The Labor Bag:

So, what shouldn't you pack? Well, as a general rule, avoid packing anything that is irreplaceable or would cause great distress if it were soiled or lost. Other than that, avoid packing things that you just won't need. Here are a few of the more common items to avoid:

1. **Underwear:** Forget about bringing your finest underwear. First of all, nobody is looking at your undies, and second, labor and delivery is a messy process. Plus, the hospital/birthing center will provide you with all of the mesh underwear that you need, and while they are not stylish, they are functional.

2. **Toiletries:** The birthing facility will likely provide you with soap, lotion, toothpaste/toothbrush, deodorant, etc. If you have a special brand that you like or if you need something hypoallergenic, you may want to bring your own.

3. **Sanitary pads:** Don't even waste your time bringing these. Not only will the hospital provide them for you, but in reality, there is probably nothing in your medicine cabinet that will even come close to what you will need after delivery.

4. **Diapers:** The hospital will provide the baby with diapers for the stay and usually a few extra to go home with, so leave the newborn diapers at home.

5. **Bottles and Formula:** If you are choosing to bottle-feed, the birthing facility will provide you with all of the formula and bottles that you need during your stay.

6. **Onesies/clothing for baby during the stay:** These will be provided by the hospital so don't waste room in your bag packing these.

7. **Baby toiletries:** Again, the birthing facility will provide things like soap and lotion for the baby, so leave yours are home.

6). And what about the car seat?

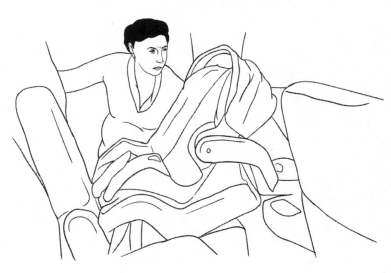

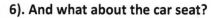

Getting the Car Ready:

Now that your bag is packed and your head is bursting with all that new found birthing class knowledge, the last thing that you have to do is get the car ready. As simple a task as this may seem, there are a few things to remember to make that day go as smoothly as possible.

1. **Car Seat:** Make sure the car seat has been placed in the car and that it is placed properly. Car seats can be deceptively tricky, and putting them in correctly may take more time than anticipated. If in doubt, many local fire departments and police stations will help with proper placement, so if you are unsure, ask for help.

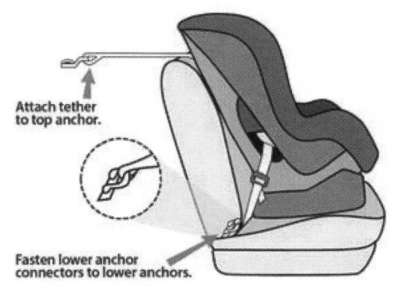

Most car seats use the LATCH (Lower Anchors and Tethers for Children) system.

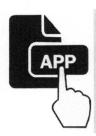

Be sure to check out the LATCH system car seat installation video in the Getting Ready for Delivery section of the app.

If you are not sure about how to install your car seat, call your local police or fire station to see which one provides a free placement service.

2. **Put the bag in the car:** Once the bag is packed, make sure that you actually put it in the trunk of the car. A well-packed bag is useless if it is sitting in your bedroom or garage when you are at the hospital or birthing center.

3. **Gas up:** Make sure you keep at least a half tank of gas in your car at all times. Imagine having to look for an open gas station at 3 AM while all the joys of labor are happening in the passenger seat.

CHAPTER 21

HOW WILL I KNOW WHEN I AM IN LABOR?

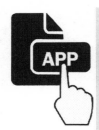 Don't forget to download the Everything Pregnancy app!

1). So, what is labor, technically?

So, how will I know when I'm actually in labor?

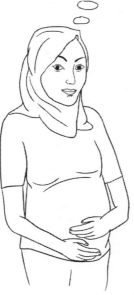

The Definition of Labor

You've been waiting a really long time for the big day to come, nine months to be exact, so you will obviously know when that time comes, right? Well, not always. We all know that everything in Hollywood is so realistic and true to life, but when it comes to labor, the woman who at one moment is happily having a nice dinner and the next is wailing in pain as her water breaks, well that just isn't reality. Nope, labor is a very gradual process, and it usually has been occurring for quite some time before you are sure that you are actually in labor.

Well, let's start with what labor actually is. This may seem like a pretty straightforward thing, but sometimes figuring out when labor has begun is not always as easy as you might think. *The technical definition of labor is regular, painful uterine contractions that cause the cervix to thin out and dilate.*

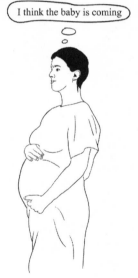

Labor is rarely like what you see in movies or on TV; it doesn't just hit you from nowhere.

How can I differentiate labor contractions from practice contractions (Braxton-Hicks)? You will have practice contractions (Braxton-Hicks) for weeks, if not months, leading up to your due date, so by the time labor actually starts, contractions will likely be nothing new to you.

So, how can you differentiate labor contractions from Braxton-Hicks contractions? Well, labor contractions:

1. Will not go away. Braxton-Hicks contractions, on the other hand, will wane with time, usually over an hour or two.

2. Will get stronger with time while Braxton-Hicks contractions are inconsistent with some stronger while others are weaker.

3. Will get closer together. Initially, labor contractions will be far apart (i.e., they may start out every 20 minutes). As labor progresses and the contractions are getting stronger, they will also get closer and closer together, eventually reaching the point where they are coming every 2-3 minutes.

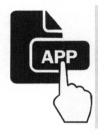

When you are ready to time your contractions, be sure to check out the Contraction Timer feature of the app.

2). Let's just keep it simple; what are the signs that labor might actually be starting?

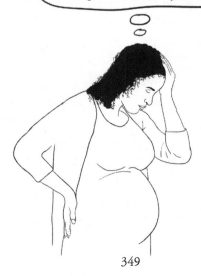

So, just break it down for me, what are the signs that I am likely in labor?

The Signs of Labor

If you are experiencing these signs, you are probably in labor:

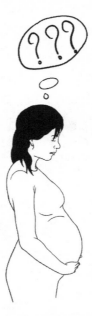

1. **Contractions that are regular and closer together,** unlike Braxton-Hicks contractions, which are irregular. Labor contractions will initially be far apart, but as you time them, they will be both regular, meaning that you can predict when the next contraction will come, and getting closer together.

2. **Contractions will become progressively more painful:** Braxton-Hicks contractions will at times be uncomfortable, but they shouldn't be painful. Labor contractions will initially be mildly uncomfortable, but as time goes on, they will get more and more painful as they get closer and closer together.

3. **Bloody Show:** Bloody show, which is a bloody mucous discharge, is a sign that the cervix is starting to dilate and thin out. It is frequently a sign of labor, especially when it is associated with contractions that are regular, getting stronger, and getting closer together. Remember, anytime you have bleeding or bloody discharge, you should call your provider, or go directly to your hospital or birthing center.

4. **Leakage of fluid:** People imagine that there will be a geyser flowing from between their legs when their bag of water breaks, and while this does make for great television, this only happens in 10% of pregnancies. Usually, when the bag of water breaks, there is a subtle, intermittent trickle of fluid that many mommies-to-be have difficulty distinguishing from urine. Anytime that you are leaking fluid from the vagina, even if it is a slow, intermittent trickle of fluid, this is likely your bag of water, and you should call your provider, and go to the hospital or birthing center immediately.

5. **Decreased fetal movement:** Many mothers report a decrease in baby's movements in the hours before labor, and while this is usually a normal occurrence before labor, if there is ever a decrease in fetal movement (either the frequency of movement or strength of movement), we recommend that you immediately perform kick counts and call your medical provider. Instructions for performing kick counts can be found in Chapter 23.

TO DO LIST

Tip for daily living: Go for stronger flavors and try adding a touch of ginger.

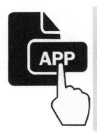

If you feel that your baby is moving less than normal, use the Fetal Kick Counter app function to keep track of your baby's movements.

6. **GI symptoms:** For many women, certain gastrointestinal symptoms can be a sign that labor is on the horizon; these include:

   ♦ *Diarrhea* or more frequent bowel movements.

   ♦ *Constipation* as the baby descends into the birth canal, putting more pressure on the colon and rectum.

- ◆ *Nausea/vomiting* (sorry, that old friend from the first trimester frequently makes a reappearance in that last lap of pregnancy).

- ◆ *Heartburn/Acid Reflux.* For many mommies-to-be acid reflux may get a little better in the last few weeks of pregnancy as the baby drops into the birth canal, relieving pressure on the stomach. As you approach labor though, it may also make an unwelcome reappearance.

7. **Vaginal/pelvic/rectal pressure:** The primary purpose of labor is for the uterus to contract, pushing your little bundle of joy down onto your cervix, causing the cervix to thin and dilate over time. As this happens, you will feel more and more pelvic and vaginal pressure, possibly accompanied by rectal pressure. While all of these are normal sensations, when you start to feel rectal pressure, it's probably a good idea to give your provider a call since this symptom tends to occur later in the labor process and could indicate that delivery is near.

3). I'm pretty sure this is labor, what the heck should I do now?!

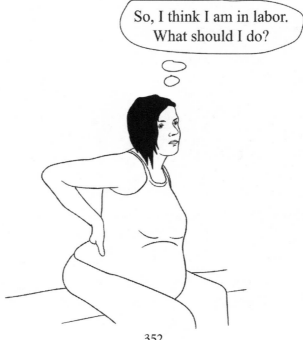

What to do When Labor Begins.

The first thing to do is take a deep breath; gather your thoughts and your remaining belongings, congratulate yourself on a pregnancy well done, and head to the hospital or birthing center to bring it all home. You have made it to the last lap of this amazing adventure, but there is still a wee bit of work ahead of you.

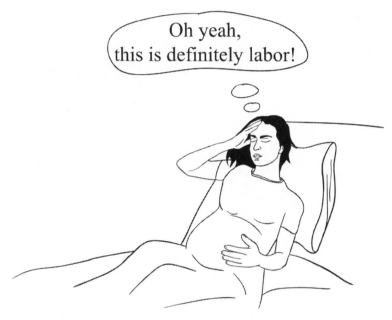

1. **Call:** Every provider will have his or her own preference, but most will want you to page them or their on-call partner to let them know that you are going to the hospital or birthing center.

2. **Support person:** Inform your support person, and make sure that he or she is in a condition to drive you.

3. **Transportation:** If your support person is not with you or is unable to drive you, either call someone nearby who can drive you or call emergency services (911/999), especially if you think that delivery is imminent.

4. **Make sure that the car is packed:** In your haste to get to the hospital or birthing center, make sure that everything on your hospital list has been packed in the car.

5. **Don't eat:** Wait until you get to the hospital or birthing center first. You need to be evaluated and given the go-ahead by your provider before you eat. If there is the possibility that a C-section may be required, you do not want to eat or drink anything beforehand.

6. **Hospital/Birthing center:** Go to the hospital/birthing center.

4). When should I definitely call my doctor or midwife?

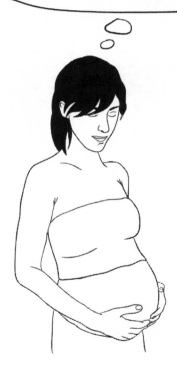

If I suspect that I am in labor, when should I call my provider?

Potentially Emergent Reasons to Call Your Medical Provider

When it comes to possible labor, these are events that should prompt you to call your provider and go immediately to the hospital or birthing center. A lot of this will be covered in Chapter 23, but here is a summary for quick reference:

1. **Decreased or no fetal movement,** especially if you weren't feeling the number of kicks that should be present while doing kick counts.

2. **Leakage of fluid vaginally:** It doesn't matter if there is a large gush or a little trickle; any leakage of fluid from the vagina warrants a visit to the hospital or birthing center.

3. **Vaginal bleeding:** While bleeding can be a normal sign of labor, any bleeding at least warrants a call to your provider.

4. **Constant or frequent abdominal pain:** Even if you don't think you are having "contractions" if your abdomen hurts continuously or frequently, you should seek medical care.

5. **Constant uterine tightness:** If your uterus or abdomen continuously or frequently feel hard, even if there is no pain, you should seek medical care.

CHAPTER 22

THE DELIVERY

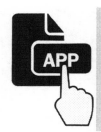 Don't forget to download the Everything Pregnancy app!

1). Okay, so it's go time! Tell me all about labor.

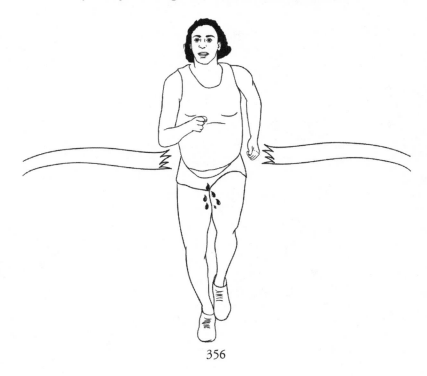

The Stages of Labor

So, what are the Stages of Labor anyway? Yes, labor has stages and phases. Who knew having a baby could be so complicated, right? Well, these are really just academic distinctions, and while it is useful information to have, knowing it will not make or break your experience.

1). First Stage of Labor: The first stage of labor is the longest stage, beginning with latent labor (early labor) and going through active labor all the way until your cervix is 10cm dilated and it is time to push.

    a. **Latent Labor** is labor, so the contractions are strong enough to cause the cervix to soften, thin, and dilate, but the contractions are not as painful or regular as they will be in active labor. Latent labor can occur for anywhere from hours to days before you enter active labor. Contractions during latent labor are more regular (so they can be timed and are predictable) than Braxton-Hicks contractions and they are definitely perceptible (unlike many Braxton-H

Exactly when latent labor ends and active labor begins is difficult to determine, but the textbook definition (ahem, we are putting on our professorial spectacles) is that latent labor becomes active labor when you reach 4 centimeters of cervical dilation. Okay, okay, we can hear you now; "How the heck will I know when I am 4cm dilated?!" The simple answer is that you won't. This is why we recommend that you contact your provider, or just go directly to the hospital or birthing center when contractions are:

1. Regular: Your contractions are coming every 8-10 minutes apart or less.
2. Painful: You can't walk or talk through them.
3. Predictable: You can predict when the next contraction will come with your good ole' contraction timer.

b. Active Labor starts at about 4cm of cervical dilation, and it occurs when contractions are painful, regular, and causing the cervix to dilate about 1 centimeter every hour. To keep it simple, by the time you hit active labor, your contractions will be very regular, very predictable, and more painful.

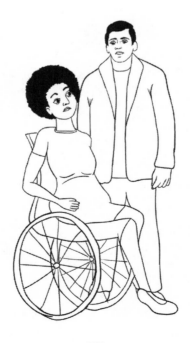

c. Transition Phase is the final part of labor when your cervix is approaching the point when it is completely dilated. Again, every pregnancy and labor is different, but generally, transition phase begins at about 8cm of dilation. Once you enter the transition phase, your labor tends to progress more quickly. During the transition phase, you will likely experience more discomfort and pressure as the contractions intensify, and the baby starts to descend into the pelvis. If you have not made your way to the hospital or birthing center by now, this would be a good time to do so.

2). Second Stage of Labor: The second stage of labor starts once your cervix is completely dilated (10cm) and continues until you deliver your bundle of joy.

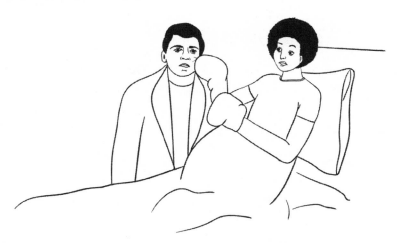

3). Third Stage of Labor: The third stage of labor starts after you deliver your baby and ends once you deliver the placenta. While placental delivery can be uncomfortable, it is nothing compared to the baby that preceded it, and many women express physical relief once the placenta is delivered.

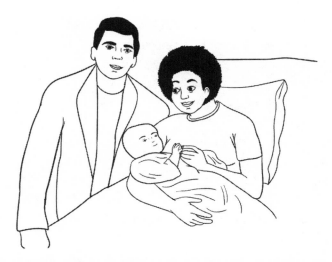

So, when the heck should I actually call my provider? Every provider is different, so be sure to ask for her or his preference, but here are some hard and fast signs that you should either reach out to your provider or just head into the hospital or birthing center:

1. Decreased fetal movement.

2. Contractions that are painful, regular, and predictable, especially if they stop you in your tracks or you have to breathe through them.

3. Any spotting or bleeding.

4. Leakage of fluid from the vagina (clear, green, or brown).

If you are a higher risk pregnancy, you may want to contact your provider earlier. **Some situations in which you should seek advice/help sooner include:**

1. Previous C-section. If you delivered by C-section in the past, your provider may not want you to labor at home for too long because of potential risks for you and baby.

2. Placental issues like a placenta previa.

3. High blood pressure/preeclampsia.

4. Multiple gestations (twin or triplet pregnancy).

5. Prior surgery on the uterus like a *myomectomy* (fibroid removal).

6. Pregnancy less than 37 weeks.

7. A baby that is not in the head down position.

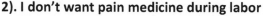

2). I don't want pain medicine during labor

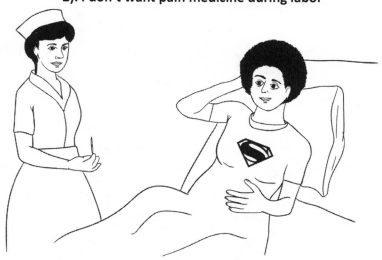

Laboring Without Pain Medication:

Hello, yes, this is very possible. Every woman's pregnancy and birth experience is her own, and there is no right or wrong way to do it. If you are opting for labor without pain medication, just know that you are joining the billions of women since time immemorial who have done the same thing. Okay, we hear you, that sounds all well and good, **but what are some real-life options that will help you achieve a labor and delivery free of pain medication? Well, here are a few to consider:**

Water labor and Water birth: Water has an anti-gravitational effect that can work wonders in reducing the pain of labor and delivery. Many hospitals and birthing centers have tubs explicitly designed for this purpose, so just ask. If this is an option you choose, make sure your birthing partner comes prepared with swimwear.

TO DO LIST

TO DO

Don't forget to pack for a pool party. Be sure to bring:

#1). A sports bra and bottoms for mom.

#2). Swimwear for partner.

#3). Towels.

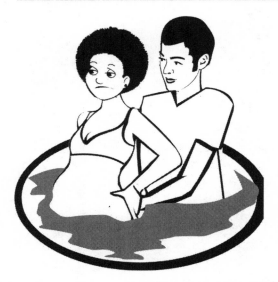

Birthing ball: Yep, they make a ball for that. The birthing ball is a large plastic ball that allows laboring moms to safely roll while sitting. This helps tilt the pelvis into more comfortable positions while also allowing the body to work with gravity.

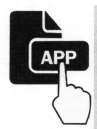

APP

Curious about how the birthing ball works? Check out the birthing ball video in the Getting Ready for Delivery section of the app.

Peanut Ball: This is a peanut-shaped ball that can be placed between the legs while you labor if you choose to labor in the bed. It has been shown to hasten labor by opening the pelvis while simultaneously relieving some of the discomforts of labor.

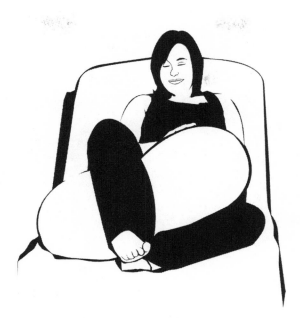

Keep it movin': Many women report that they feel less pain during labor if they are mobile. You will have to find your sweet spot, but many mothers find it most comfortable to walk between contractions while stopping to either rock back and forth or bend forward during a contraction. If you and your baby have to be monitored continuously, see if your hospital or birthing center offers walking monitors.

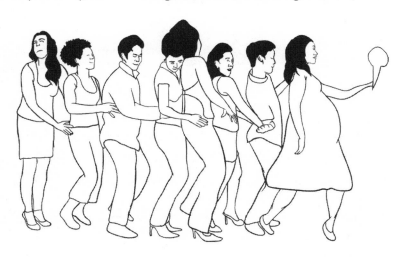

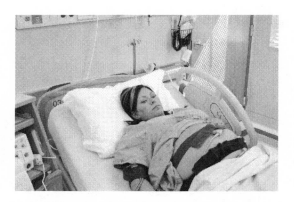

Most fetal heart rate/contraction monitors are stationary.

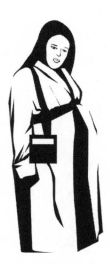

A walking monitor can monitor the baby and your contractions while allowing you to be mobile.

Warm Shower: There is nothing like a nice warm shower to soothe the lower back pain that frequently accompanies labor. Just make sure you have someone with you to help keep you steady and balanced.

Assume the position: And by this, we mean any safe position that you want to assume. Every mommy-to-be is different, and the position you find most comfortable will likely be unique to you. Some women like to lie flat on their back in bed, while others prefer to lie on their sides. Many women prefer laboring while on their hands and knees or even squatting. Don't be shy; this is your show, and you are free to experiment with positions as long as your provider feels that it is safe.

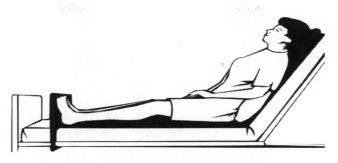

Some women labor lying in bed on their backs.

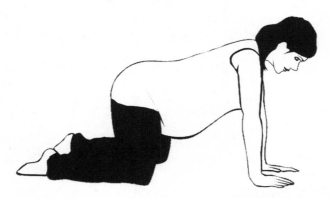

Laboring in the hands-knees position may help reduce lower back discomfort.

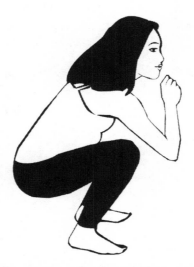

Frequent squatting will reduce pelvic pressure while allowing gravity to help dilate the cervix.

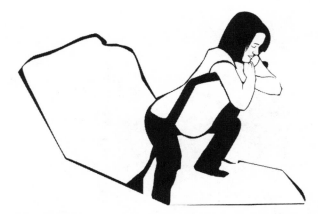

A squat bar helps to mimic the squatting position for women confined to the bed (think women with an epidural).

TO DO LIST

If you are bed bound, be sure to ask about using the squatting bar.

Hypno-birthing: Yes, this is an actual thing, and no, it is not restricted to sunny California. Many women report great success when it comes to relieving labor pain with hypnosis. If you can train your mind to stop smoking, why can't you train it to feel less pain during labor and delivery?

Doula: A doula is a person who specializes in attending to the physical and emotional needs of laboring mothers and their families. The duties of a doula range from massage, to helping with breathing, to serving as emotional support for the entire team.

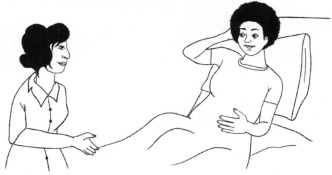

Breathing: There are a multitude of breathing techniques that can help during labor, and your provider or prenatal educator may have a technique that they prefer. One technique that we have found works well involves taking slow deep breaths through your nose as the contraction begins and then slowly exhaling through your mouth when the contraction reaches maximal intensity. Most women close their eyes and focus on a specific part of their body (other than their uterus) while doing this. Many women will also picture riding the contraction like a wave as they deep breathe.

Acupressure: Not only can acupressure do wonders for pain relief during labor, but some studies suggest that it can speed the process up as well.

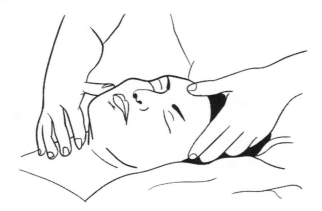

Many women report that acupressure helps to reduce the pain and anxiety of labor.

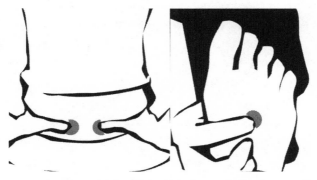

Specific pressure points have also been found to help with labor progression.

Meditation: Meditation is all about centering yourself, and there are meditation classes designed specifically for labor and delivery that many women find helpful.

Massage: A good focused massage, especially of the lower back, can feel like a little slice of heaven, especially if you are experiencing back labor.

3). What are my pain medication options during labor?

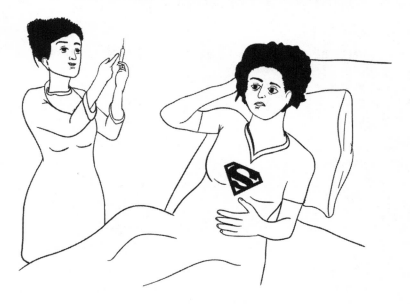

Laboring with Pain Medication:

In case you haven't figured it out yet, any woman who has the strength to carry and nurture a life under her heart for nine months is a superwoman, and the decision to use or forego pain medication during labor doesn't change that one little bit. So, if you are considering pain medications during labor, what are your options?

IV Narcotics: IV Narcotics include medications like Stadol, Demerol, and Morphine which are given through the IV to reduce pain and anxiety during labor. While these medications will blunt some of the pain and help you to relax, they will not completely take the pain away, and you will still experience some discomfort.

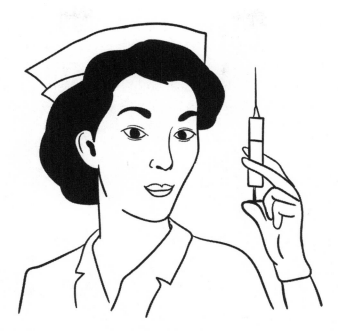

1. **PROS:** They are easy to administer and relatively non-invasive.

2. **CONS:** Do not completely relieve pain, and if given within a couple of hours of delivery, they can make the baby a bit sluggish, and in some cases, slow his or her breathing. If this occurs, there are medications that easily reverse this side effect.

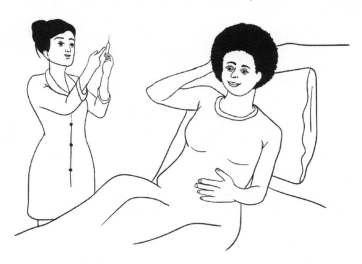

Laughing Gas: Laughing gas, aka nitrous oxide, is not just for the dentist. Laughing gas, as the name suggests, is given in inhalation form, and more and more hospitals are using it for laboring mothers. Despite the name, it likely won't have you giggling your labor away, but it does help to reduce anxiety while also providing some pain relief.

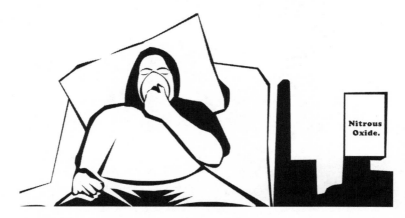

1. **PROS:** Easy to administer, no effects on the baby, relieves anxiety.

2. **CONS:** Relieves pain minimally, can cause some nausea.

Old Wives Tale

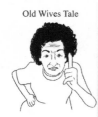

"Laughing gas makes you high and giggly!" Despite the name, laughing gas doesn't always make you laugh or giggle.

Epidural: Epidural is the most common form of pain relief during labor. The epidural process involves placing a small catheter (think of a very small, flexible tube) into *the epidural space* above the nerves in the spinal cord. Medication is then delivered through this catheter, bathing the nerves, causing numbness from about the level of the belly button down. The epidural effect is pretty rapid, kicking in within 10-20 minutes. Despite common misconception, there is no best time to get the epidural, and you don't have to wait a certain amount of time before you can get it. When you feel like you need it, you ask for it.

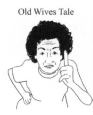

"Don't get an epidural unless you want to be paralyzed": Despite the common concern that an epidural can cause paralysis, the risk of paralysis after an epidural is about 0.00001%

1. **PROS:** Provides complete or near complete pain relief.

2. **CONS:** Restricts you to the bed usually; invasive with some discomfort during placement; can sometimes cause an intense headache called a spinal headache, which is treated with fluids, pain medications, rest, and tincture of time.

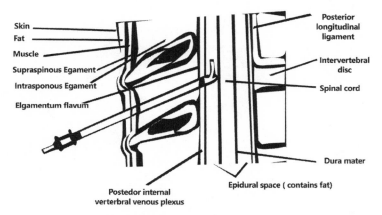

The epidural catheter is a small tube that goes in to a space called the epidural space, delivering medication that numbs the nerves.

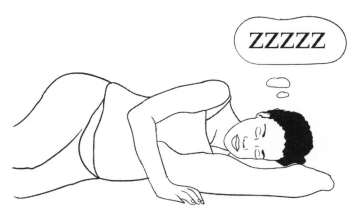

The single biggest benefit of an epidural is comfort and the ability to rest.

Local pain medications: Local pain medications, like Lidocaine, are numbing medicines that are injected into the perineum (the area between the vagina and anus) or the vagina. While these will provide some pain relief during the actual delivery phase, they become more necessary if you do not have an epidural, and your provider is going to cut an episiotomy, or if you tear and they need to sew the tear.

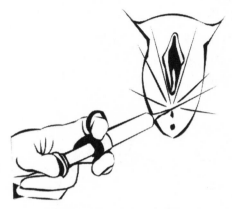

The injection of the numbing medication burns but this is only momentary.

4). Okay, I just have to ask. Is it true that *other* things can come out during labor and delivery?

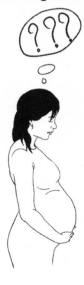

Urination, Bowel Movements, and Vomiting During Labor.

Labor and delivery are natural processes, and what's more natural than the most primal bodily functions, right? Many mommies-to-be find it surprising that urination, defecation, and vomiting are pretty common parts of labor and delivery. As embarrassing as this may sound, just know that it is totally normal; it happens to many women, and your healthcare team has seen it thousands of times before.

Urination: Many women do empty their bladder during the second stage of labor when they are pushing; it's just a fact of life. Let's be honest folks, the bladder and uterus live in the same neighborhood, and what affects one will frequently affect the other. While most of your pushing will be directed towards your uterus, some of it will also reach the bladder, resulting in loss of urine. If you have an epidural, a Foley catheter will likely be placed to drain the bladder, in which case you will not have to worry about urinating. So, what can you do to reduce the likelihood of urinating during the second stage of labor? If you don't have an epidural and a Foley catheter, you can attempt to empty your bladder using a bedpan or the toilet before you start pushing.

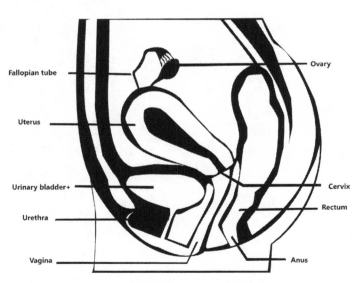

The uterus is close to the bladder, and as it contracts during labor, it puts a great deal of pressure on the bladder.

Defecation: For all the same reasons that you might urinate during the second stage of labor, you can also have a bowel movement. The uterus and the rectum are also in the same neighborhood, and once again, some of the force directed towards the uterus will naturally reach your rectum. In fact, many moms will tell you that the pressure experienced during delivery feels very much like the pressure of having a bowel movement. Much like urinating during the second stage, having a bowel movement is completely normal, and it happens way more often than you would think. So, what can you do to possibly avoid this? Emptying your bowels before you hit active labor is the best thing, but make sure your provider checks the cervix before doing so as many a woman has mistaken a baby for a bowel movement and delivered on the toilet. Some folks will use an enema when labor starts, but this really isn't necessary. So, if it does happen, don't be embarrassed, and know that your healthcare team has experienced this many, many times in the past.

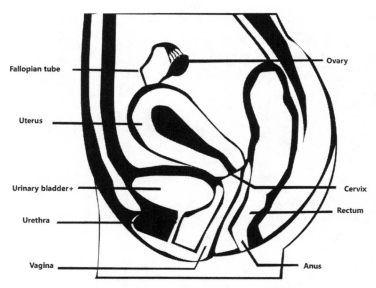

*Much like the bladder, the growing uterus presses
on the intestines, especially during labor.*

Vomiting: Vomiting during labor and delivery also definitely happens. Between the hormonal fluctuations that occur and the pain that you can experience, many women do vomit during both labor as well as delivery. This most commonly happens during the second phase, when you are pushing. There really is no good way to avoid this, but some providers will restrict eating and drinking during labor to reduce the risk of vomiting. In most cases, there is no need to restrict food and drink during labor, but we do recommend keeping things light and high in protein to build up that energy. If nausea does rear its ugly head, your provider can likely give you medications to reduce nausea and vomiting, so be sure to ask.

5). Okay, let's talk about this ring of fire.

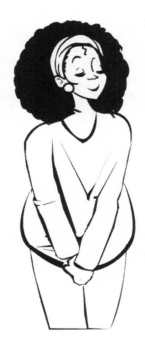

Delivery and The Ring of Fire.

Yup, it is a thing. The ring of fire is a very descriptive term for what your vagina and perineum (the area between the vagina and anus) may feel like at the moment your bundle of joy is crowning. *Crowning* is the term for when the largest diameter of your baby's head is being delivered. Because this is the point at which the vagina and perineum are being most stretched, this is the most uncomfortable part of the delivery. This stretching produces an intense burning sensation that is aptly called the ring of fire. Many women that have an epidural experience a much less intense ring of fire or feel nothing at all. The ring of fire is generally most intense with your first delivery, though it will be present for every delivery.

If you don't have an epidural, what are some things that you can do to reduce the intensity of the ring of fire?

1. **Perineal massage** using lubricants (olive oil, water-based lubricant, etc.) before and during labor will ready the skin for stretching.

TO DO LIST

TO DO

This may sound a bit strange, but start to massage and gently stretch your perineum a couple of times per day starting at 36 weeks. Before doing so, be sure to get the okay from your medical provider. Olive oil or vegetable oil are both relatively cheap and easy to use for these massages.

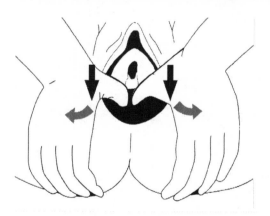

Gently massage the lower portion of the vaginal opening from the 3 o'clock to 9 o'clock positions.

2. **Controlled delivery of the head** by reducing your pushing force during crowning can lessen the crowning intensity and the likelihood of experiencing a tear.

3. **Perineal support by your delivery provider** prevents the perineum from over-stretching and potentially tearing during crowning.

4. **Water births** can reduce the effect of gravity and the ring of fire.

5. **Delivering in a semi-reclined position.**

Baby crowning

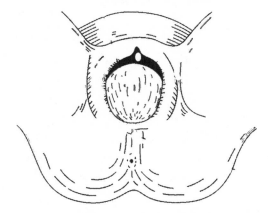

Crowning occurs when the maximum diameter of the baby's head is passing the vaginal opening.

Just remember why you are doing this

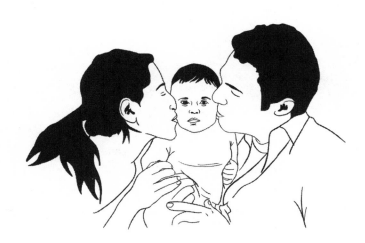

CHAPTER 23

WHEN IS IT TIME TO CALL YOUR PROVIDER? PREGNANCY WARNING SIGNS AND COMPLICATIONS

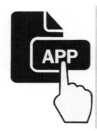 **Don't forget to download the Everything Pregnancy app!**

1). What are the important signs and symptoms that I need to watch for?

Potential Pregnancy Warning Signs:

You will experience a myriad of symptoms from the start of your pregnancy to the end, and every trimester comes with its own potential problems and complications. Rest assured that the majority of pregnancies go off without a hitch, but there are situations that warrant you reaching out to your provider. What follows is a pretty comprehensive list of those times, but if you have a symptom or concern that is not on this list, you should always reach out to your provider. *Experiencing one of these symptoms does not necessarily mean doom or gloom, but it does mean that you should reach out and get in touch with someone.* Your provider and her or his team are there for this reason and should be available to you 24-7.

VAGINAL BLEEDING: Many women will experience vaginal spotting or bleeding at some point during a healthy pregnancy, so fear not. However, if you have experienced vaginal spotting or bleeding, you should always let your provider know. For more information, please check out the section on spotting/bleeding in Chapter 9.

Old Wives Tale

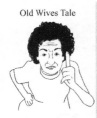

"It's okay to bleed during pregnancy": Bleeding during pregnancy should never be seen as normal until your provider rules out more serious conditions. There is no such a thing as still having your period while you are pregnant.

SEVERE CRAMPING OR ABDOMINAL PAIN: Most pregnant women will experience cramping and bloating. In fact, many mommies-to-be report that they frequently feel like their period is going to start. While cramping is normal, it can be more concerning if:

1. It is severe, persistent, or regularly consistent.

2. It is one-sided.

3. It is associated with a fever.

4. It is associated with diarrhea.

5. It is associated with spotting or bleeding.

PASSAGE OF CLOTS OR TISSUE FROM THE VAGINA: Anytime there is bleeding, clots can form. Clots, however, tend to indicate heavier bleeding and are therefore a bit more concerning. You should let your provider know if you pass clots or tissue at any time but especially if:

1. It is associated with cramping or pelvic pain.

2. The associated bleeding is heavy.

3. It is associated with leakage of fluid from the vagina.

SEVERE DIZZINESS OR PASSING OUT: While some dizziness during pregnancy can be normal, symptoms that are persistent or debilitating should be reported to your provider. For more information, check out Chapter 11.

SEVERE NAUSEA/VOMITING: The vast majority of pregnant women will experience some nausea and/or vomiting during pregnancy, especially in the first trimester. For more information on nausea/vomiting, be sure to check out Chapter 6. While nausea during pregnancy is normal, you should reach out to your provider if you are experiencing any of the following:

1. Persistent vomiting with the inability to hold anything down for more than 24-hours.

2. Symptoms of dehydration like dry mouth, concentrated urine, or dizziness.

3. The nausea is associated with severe diarrhea and/or fever.

4. The nausea/vomiting is associated with headache.

Old Wives Tale

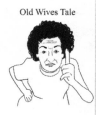

"You just have to live with nausea and vomiting during pregnancy": Severe or persistent nausea and vomiting is not just "something you have to deal with." Your provider has a lot of options to reduce nausea and vomiting, helping you return to a relatively normal life.

PAINFUL URINATION: Every mommy-to-be is going to spend a lot of time in the bathroom. A growing uterus pressing on the bladder means lots of trips to the bathroom. While frequent urination is completely normal, urination should not be painful, and if it is, you should reach out to your provider, especially if it is associated with:

1. Fevers and/or chills.

2. Back pain (especially on just one side).

LEAKAGE OF FLUID FROM THE VAGINA: Vaginas will make more discharge during pregnancy; that is a normal and actually protective response. For more information, check out Chapter 9. There are times, however, when leakage or drainage from the vagina is not normal, including if the discharge:

1. Is copious.

2. Is clear and watery or has a green or brown color.

3. Has a foul odor.

4. Is associated with spotting, bleeding, cramping, or contractions.

A CHANGE IN YOUR BABY'S MOVEMENTS: By 20-24 weeks of pregnancy, most babies will have movement patterns. Some babies move all day long, while others are more active only at certain times of the day. Be sure to check out the section in Chapter 2 discussing Kick Counts, what they are, and how to do them. Get to know your baby's patterns, and if they change in any way, you should reach out to your provider ASAP, especially if you experience any of the following:

1. A noticeable decrease in the frequency and/or intensity of the baby's movements.

2. Inadequate fetal kick counts.

3. Contractions, cramping, spotting, or bleeding associated with a decrease in fetal movement.

Old Wives Tale

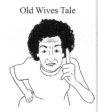

"If your baby doesn't move, s/he is probably just lazy": There is no such a thing as a lazy baby. Know your baby's patterns, and if they change or reduce, don't chalk it up to a lazy baby.

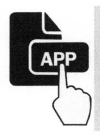

Be sure to use the app's Kick Counter to monitor your baby's movement.

SEVERE OR PERSISTENT HEADACHES: Headaches during pregnancy are also quite common thanks to those lovely hormones. For more information about headaches and pregnancy, please be sure to check out Chapter 11. While usually normal, you should contact your provider if your headaches are:

1. Severe and persistent.

2. Associated with dizziness or loss of consciousness.

3. Associated with persistent vomiting.

4. Associated with visual changes or blurry vision.

5. Associated with cramping, contractions, or abdominal pain.

VISUAL CHANGES: Now, we already know that pregnancy is a total body experience, and even your vision will be affected. For more details about vision during pregnancy, be sure to check out Chapter 4. There are times, however, when visual changes should be reported to your provider, and these include:

1. Sudden onset or severe visual changes.

2. Visual changes associated with a headache, dizziness, or loss of consciousness.

3. Visual changes associated with abdominal pain.

LEG PAIN OR SWELLING: Pregnancy and swollen legs go together like peanut butter and jelly (if you don't believe us, be sure to check out Chapter 15), but there are times when symptoms in your legs could be potentially dangerous. If you experience any of the following, you should reach out to your provider:

1. Sudden onset or severe swelling, especially if it involves just one side.

2. Redness or heat radiating from one or both legs.

3. Pain with walking or when you flex the leg.

CHEST PAIN/SHORTNESS OF BREATH: While mild shortness of breath is normal during pregnancy (for full details be sure to check out Chapter 7), you should contact your provider ASAP if you experience any of the following:

1. Chest pain with or without exertion.

2. Sudden onset of shortness of breath.

3. Cough, especially with mucus production.

4. A drowning or choking sensation when you lie flat.

5. Fever.

6. Wheezing.

EXTREME SWELLING: Swelling in the lower and upper extremities during pregnancy is normal (check out Chapter 14 for more information), but you should contact your provider if you experience any of the following:

1. Sudden onset or extreme swelling.
2. Swelling that is significantly more pronounced on only one side.
3. Swelling associated with redness, warmth, or pain in the limb.
4. Headache and/or visual changes with the swelling.

FEVER: Fevers are a normal bodily response to infection, and they actually serve an essential function. Temperatures above a certain level, however, can pose a danger to pregnancy, especially in the first trimester, so you should reach out to your provider if:

1. You experience a fever over 102.5 degrees Fahrenheit.

DEPRESSION: A little sadness every now and again is a normal part of life, especially during times of stress, and the hormones associated with pregnancy (and post-partum) will only compound this. For more information, be sure to check out Chapter 18. There is, however, a line between normal sadness and depression, and you should reach out to your provider if you experience:

1. Sudden onset of sadness.
2. Severe sadness that inhibits your ability to get through your day normally.
3. Sleep changes, either sleeping too much or insomnia.
4. Loss of interest in things that generally interest you.
5. Lots of crying.
6. Sudden loss of energy, motivation, or concentration.
7. Feelings of guilt.

*****If you have thoughts of harming yourself or harming others, you should seek immediate emergency care.*****

***** If you hear voices or see things that are not there, you should seek immediate emergency care.*****

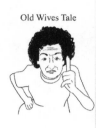
"Of course you are depressed honey, you are pregnant": It is not normal to be depressed during pregnancy. Feeling blue from time to time, especially after baby comes can be normal, but depression is not. If you are experiencing symptoms of depression, reach out to your provider ASAP!

ITCHING: A little itch here or there is totally normal, but there are times when itching during pregnancy can be abnormal (see Cholestasis of Pregnancy in chapter 3 and below), and you should reach out to your provider if you experience any of the following:

1. Itching that is worse after a warm bath or shower.

2. Itching associated with a rash, especially on the abdomen.

3. Itching that is intense and primarily involves the palms of the hands and the soles of the feet.

What are some things that can go wrong?

Common Pregnancy-Related Complications:

CERVICAL INSUFFICIENCY: Also known as *cervical incompetence*, this is a condition in which the cervix prematurely (usually between 13-24 weeks of pregnancy) and painlessly thins out (effaces) and dilates. Patient's with cervical insufficiency will often experience perfuse watery discharge, pelvic pressure, and finally premature breaking of the bag of water. Evidence of cervical insufficiency can be detected on ultrasound, and a stitch called a *cerclage* can be placed in the cervix to prevent further dilation and thinning in the current pregnancy, as well as future pregnancies. Women have a greater risk of developing cervical insufficiency if they have had it in a prior pregnancy or if they have had any surgeries on their cervix.

Normal cervix   Incompetent Cervix

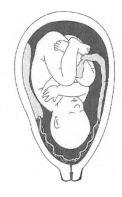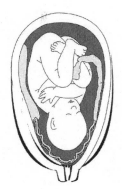

*Cervical incompetence (or insufficiency) is marked by
a cervix that thins and dilates too early.*

Cervical cerclage.

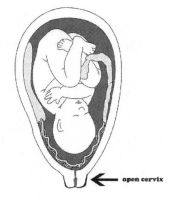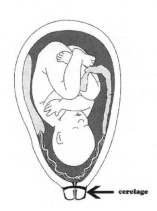

open cervix   cerclage

*A cerclage is a stitch placed in the cervix to close it,
hopefully preventing further dilation and thinning.*

CHOLESTASIS OF PREGNANCY: Women with this condition have higher than normal levels of bile acids, which are produced by the liver, in their blood. Patients with cholestasis report intense itching, especially involving the palms of the hands and the soles of the feet. There are medications that can be taken to reduce the level of bile acids and reduce itching; however, cholestasis does increase the risk of poor fetal growth and possible fetal death, which is why these pregnancies are monitored closely, and usually labor is induced a few weeks before the due date.

ECLAMPSIA: Eclampsia is a severe form of preeclampsia (high blood pressure specific to pregnancy, see below) associated with seizures. Patients with eclampsia are given medications to reduce their blood pressure as well as *magnesium sulfate*, a medication which reduces the risk of future seizures. Regardless of gestational age, if severe preeclampsia or eclampsia develops, labor is generally induced, as delivery is the only cure. Women with chronic high blood pressure or a prior history of preeclampsia or eclampsia are at a higher risk of developing this condition.

ECTOPIC PREGNANCY: This is a pregnancy that implants and grows outside of the uterus. The most common location is one of the fallopian tubes, though ectopic pregnancies can also occur on the ovaries, in the pelvis, or on the cervix. Ectopic pregnancies cannot progress to a point where the baby can live outside of the uterus, and the pregnancies must be ended either with surgery, or a medication called *methotrexate*, to save the mother's life. Women who have had a prior ectopic pregnancy or a previous infection in, or surgery on, the fallopian tubes, have a higher risk of future ectopic pregnancies.

NORMAL PREGNANCY

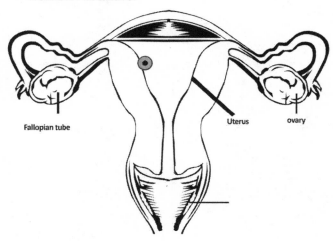

Fallopian tube

Uterus   ovary

A normal pregnancy implants higher in the uterus.

386

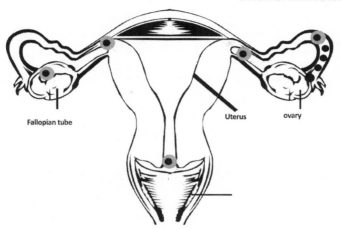

An ectopic pregnancy implants in any location other than the uterus.

GESTATIONAL DIABETES: Gestational diabetes is diabetes specific to pregnancy. Women with gestational diabetes have a higher risk of developing it again in subsequent pregnancies and also have a higher risk of developing type 2 diabetes in the future. Women who have had a prior pregnancy affected by gestational diabetes, a family history of diabetes, or who are overweight, have a higher likelihood of developing gestational diabetes. This condition can sometimes be treated with diet and exercise alone, but sometimes medications (either pills or insulin injections) are required. Mothers-to-be with gestational diabetes will need to have their babies monitored more closely, especially at the end of pregnancy.

GESTATIONAL HYPERTENSION: This is another high blood pressure condition specific to pregnancy. Hypertension is usually defined as a systolic blood pressure of 130 or more (the top number) or a diastolic blood pressure of 80 or more (the bottom number). Women with gestational hypertension are at higher risk of developing preeclampsia during pregnancy as well as hypertension when they are no longer pregnant. Gestational hypertension can sometimes be treated with just diet and exercise, but frequently, medication may also be needed. Mothers-to-be with Gestational hypertension will need to have their babies monitored more closely, especially at the end of pregnancy when complications are more likely.

HYPEREMESIS GRAVIDARUM: This is a condition characterized by severe and persistent nausea and vomiting, especially during the first trimester of pregnancy. Hyperemesis is more than just the normal nausea and vomiting of pregnancy as it can lead to severe weight loss and electrolyte disturbances. There are a multitude of medications that can be used to treat hyperemesis, and developing hyperemesis in one pregnancy increases the likelihood that you will develop it in future pregnancies. Hyperemesis is also more common in pregnancies with multiples.

INTRAUTERINE FETAL DEMISE (IUFD): IUFD is the term used for the death of a baby while still in the uterus. The likelihood of IUFD is increased in high-risk pregnancies, and while it is thankfully a rare phenomenon, many women report that a decrease in fetal movement preceded the IUFD. Women who have experienced a prior IUFD will be at higher risk in future pregnancies and therefore will have more intensive monitoring and likely earlier induction of labor.

INTRAUTERINE GROWTH RESTRICTION (IUGR): IUGR is the term given when a baby's growth is less than that expected for its gestational age. The cut-off depends upon the source you are reading, but generally, a baby at the 10th percentile or less for weight is considered *small for gestational age (SGA)* while a baby at or below the 5th percentile is considered IUGR. Both conditions are more common in mothers with chronic medical conditions, mothers over the age of 35, and mothers who smoke cigarettes. Small for gestational age and IUGR pregnancies will be monitored more closely, and they will likely be induced before their due dates.

MISCARRIAGE/SPONTANEOUS   ABORTION: A miscarriage, or spontaneous abortion is the involuntary loss of a pregnancy before 20 weeks' gestation. Many miscarriages occur before a woman even knows that she is pregnant, and almost all will occur before 10 weeks' gestation. Most miscarriages are sporadic, meaning they happen by chance, and having one does not put a woman at an increased risk of having another. There are rare situations where mothers do have a condition making them more prone to recurrent miscarriage, and it is recommended that any woman who has had two or more consecutive miscarriages be evaluated for one of these rare conditions.

MOLAR PREGNANCY: A molar pregnancy is an abnormal pregnancy that occurs when a non-viable egg is fertilized, resulting in the rapid growth of placenta-like tissue. Molar pregnancies are associated with rapid uterine growth, cramping, and bleeding, as well as exaggerated symptoms of pregnancy, including fatigue, nausea, and vomiting. Molar pregnancies are not viable, and they have to be treated by emptying the uterus of the abnormal tissue, a procedure called a D&C (dilation and curettage).

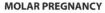

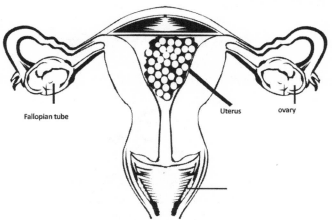

A molar pregnancy is characterized by the growth of fluid-filled vesicles in the uterus.

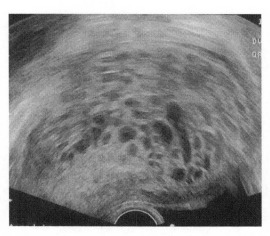

Molar pregnancies have a "snowstorm" appearance on ultrasound.

OLIGOHYDRAMNIOS: Oligohydramnios occurs when the amniotic fluid level is lower than normal (usually 5cm or less). The most common cause of oligohydramnios is leakage of amniotic fluid, but it can also be seen in other situations like poorly managed hypertension and maternal smoking.

PLACENTAL ABRUPTION: A placental abruption occurs when the placenta separates from the wall of the uterus prematurely (before birth). Placental abruptions are usually associated with cramping, frequent contractions, spotting or bleeding, and a decrease in fetal movement. Placental abruptions are more common after maternal abdominal trauma and in mothers with high blood pressure or who use cocaine. Most symptomatic cases of placental abruption, especially in term or near-term pregnancies, will require labor induction or delivery by cesarean section.

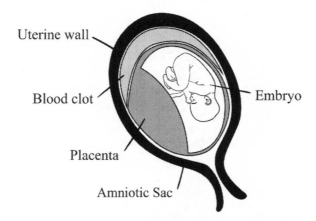

Placental abruption is the premature separation of the placenta from the wall of the uterus, frequently resulting in bleeding.

PLACENTA PREVIA: This is a condition in which the placenta covers the cervix (outlet of the uterus). The coverage can be either partial or complete. Placenta previa is more common in mothers over the age of 35, women who have had a prior placenta previa, women who have had previous uterine surgeries, including C-sections, and women who smoke. The most common symptom of a previa is bleeding, and these pregnancies have to be delivered by C-section since the cervix is blocked.

PLACENTA PREVIA

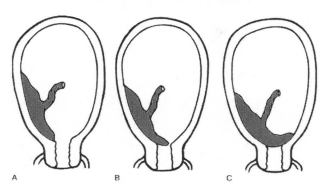

A   B   C

Placenta previa occurs when the placenta partially or completely covers the cervix.

POLYHYDRAMNIOS: Polyhydramnios is the opposite of oligohydramnios, and it occurs when there is more than the usual amount of amniotic fluid, generally 20cm or more. Polyhydramnios is most frequently seen in diabetic mothers who are not controlling their blood sugar well. Women with polyhydramnios tend to have more contractions throughout their pregnancies and also have a higher risk of the bag of water breaking before their due dates.

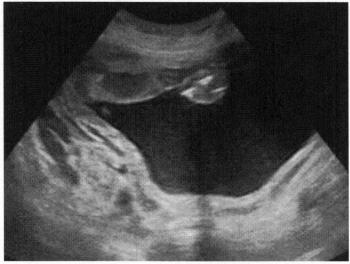

Amniotic fluid is black on ultrasound. Polyhydramnios is evident when there is an excess of this black appearing fluid.

391

PREECLAMPSIA: This is a high blood pressure condition exclusive to pregnancy. Women with preeclampsia also have increased levels of protein in their urine and have a higher risk of developing eclampsia (seizures, see above). Women with high blood pressure before pregnancy have a higher risk of preeclampsia, and having preeclampsia in one pregnancy increases the risk of developing it in future pregnancies. Other symptoms of Preeclampsia include extreme swelling, headaches, and visual changes. In pregnancies close to their due dates, or when mom's blood pressure reaches a certain threshold, labor will have to be induced as delivery is the only cure.

PREMATURE RUPTURE OF MEMBRANES: Premature rupture of membranes occurs when the bag of water breaks before labor starts. This can be before or after your due date. In most cases, labor will begin soon thereafter on its own, but in some cases, medications will have to be given to induce labor because the risk of infection increases once the bag of water breaks.

PRETERM RUPTURE OF MEMBRANES: This occurs when the bag of water breaks before the 37th week of pregnancy. If the bag of water breaks at or after 34 weeks, labor will likely be induced. If the bag of water breaks before 34 weeks, you will be given steroids to mature the baby's lungs and organs and antibiotics to prevent infection. Once you reach 34 weeks' gestation, labor will likely be induced. If infection occurs at any point, labor will have to be induced.

PRETERM LABOR: Labor that occurs before 37 weeks' gestation is known as preterm labor. Generally, preterm labor will not be stopped if it occurs after 36 weeks, while labor before 36 weeks' gestation will usually be stopped with a group of medications call *tocolytics*.

CHAPTER 24

SAFE MEDICATIONS FOR COMMON CONDITIONS

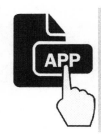 Don't forget to download the Everything Pregnancy app!

1). Aches, pains, fevers, and other ills, what can I take doc?

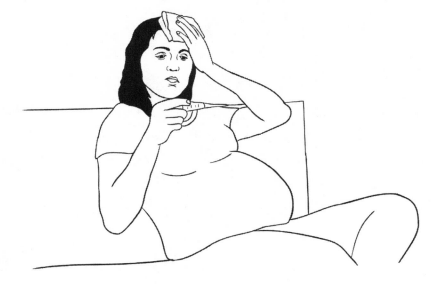

Medications Usually Considered Safe to Take During Pregnancy:

Sure, pregnancy comes with its own aches and pains, a fact with which you are likely intimately familiar by now. Not every discomfort that you experience during pregnancy is pregnancy related, however. Yup, as unfair as it might seem, being pregnant doesn't exempt you from all those other everyday conditions that can also make you miserable. So, if one of these conditions should rear its ugly head, what can you take to feel better?

In reality, there are very few medications that can be guaranteed to be 100% safe during pregnancy because pregnant women are rarely included in the studies used to determine the safety of new medications coming to market. In fact, only 10% of medications currently approved by the U.S. Food and Drug Administration (FDA) have enough information to definitively determine their risk for causing congenital disabilities. For this reason, we always recommend that you reach out to your provider before starting any new medication, even medications on this safe list. Here, however, is a list of common conditions that many women experience during pregnancy and medications that can be taken to relieve these symptoms.

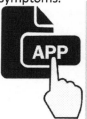

Curious if a medication is safe to use during pregnancy? Check out the FDA Medication Information feature of the app. Before you start any new medication, be sure to speak with your medical provider.

TO DO LIST

Before taking a new medication or continuing a pre-pregnancy medication, be sure to reach out to your provider first, and then check out the FDA Medication Information feature of the app.

CONDITION:	SAFE MEDICATIONS:
Aches and Pains	• Acetaminophen (Tylenol, Paracetamol).
Acne	• Benzoyl peroxide
	• Over the counter astringents
Allergies and Hay Fever	• Antihistamines including Diphenhydramine (Benadryl) and Loratadine (Claritin, Alavert)
	• Steroid Nasal Sprays (Rhinocort, Nasonex, Flonase)
	• Acetaminophen (Tylenol and Tylenol Sinus, Paracetamol)
	• Saline nasal sprays
Constipation	• Neti pot/nasal lavage
	• Fiber supplements (Citrucil, Metamucil)
	• Stool Softeners (Docusate, Colace)
	• Laxatives (Senekot, Dulcolax)
Cough and Cold Symptoms	• Milk of Magnesia
	• Acetaminophen (Tylenol and Tylenol Cold, Paracetamol)
	• Benadryl
	• Cough Drops
	• Vicks Vaporub
	• Dextromethorphan and Guaifenesin (Robitussin and Mucinex)
Minor Cuts and Scrapes	• Topical antibiotic creams and gels (Bacitracin, Neosporin, Polysporin)
Diarrhea	• Loperamide (Imodium)
	• Diphenoxylate (Lomotil)
Fever	• Bismuth (Kaopectate)
	• Acetaminophen (Tylenol or Tylenol Extra Strength, Paracetamol)

Gas Pain	• Simethicone (Mylicon, Gas-X)
Headache	• Acetaminophen (Tylenol or Tylenol Extra Strength, Paracetamol)
	• Caffeine (12oz per day or less)
Heartburn/ Reflux	• Antacids (TUMS, Maalox, Mylanta, Rolaids)
	• Acid suppressors (Zantac, Tagamet, Prilosec, Protonix)
Hemorrhoids	• Preparation H, Anusol
	• Tucks pads
	• Hydrocortisone cream or gel
Insomnia	• Diphenhydramine (Benadryl, Sominex)
	• Doxylamine (Unisom)
Itching and Rash	• Diphenhydramine (Benadryl)
	• Oatmeal Bath (Aveeno)
	• Hydrocortisone (Caladryl, Cortaid)
Nasal Congestion/ Stuffy Nose	• Antihistamines including Diphenhydramine (Benadryl) and Loratadine (Claritin, Alavert)
	• Steroid Nasal Sprays (Rhinocort, Nasonex, Flonase)
	• Acetaminophen (Tylenol and Tylenol Cold, Tylenol Sinus)
	• Vicks Vaporub
	• Dextromethorphan and Guaifenesin (Robitussin and Mucinex)
	• Saline nasal sprays
	• Neti Pot/Nasal lavage

Nausea and Vomiting	• Vitamin B6 (100mg tablets)
	• Dramamine
	• Unisom
	• Benadryl
	• Ginger root capsules (250mg four times a day)
	• Sea Bands
Pain	• Acetaminophen (Tylenol or Paracetamol)
Sore Throat	• Benzocaine/Menthol lozenges (Cepachol)
	• Benzocaine spray (Chloraseptic)
	• Warm salt water gargles
Yeast Infection	• Clotrimazole (Gyne Lotrimin)
	• Tioconazole (Monistat-1)
	• Terconazole (Terazol)
	• Miconazole (Monistat-3)

(Be careful not to insert the applicator to deep.)

2). And what about my herbs and supplements?

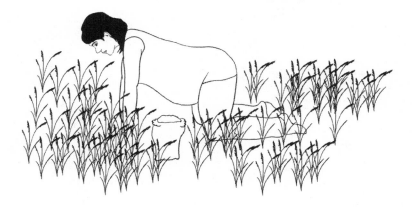

A Quick Word About Herbal Supplements During Pregnancy:

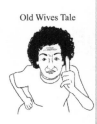

Old Wives Tale

"If it comes from the earth, it is safe": Not everything that comes from the earth or is classified as "natural" is safe for use during pregnancy. Check out the list of no-no herbal and alternative medications below, and talk to your provider before starting or continuing any herbal or alternative medication.

Not everything that comes from the earth is safe to take during pregnancy. Much like traditional medications, therefore, we recommend that you discuss any herbal medications with your provider before you start or continue taking them. Due to known risks of congenital disabilities, these herbal and alternative medications should be avoided during pregnancy:

1. Arbor Vitae.
2. Basil essential oil.
3. Beth root.
4. Black Cohosh.
5. Blue Cohosh.
6. Calamus essential oil.
7. Cascara.
8. Chaste tree berry.
9. Chinese angelica/Dong Quai.
10. Cinchona.
11. Cotton root bark.
12. Feverfew.
13. Ginseng.
14. Golden Seal.
15. Hyssop essential oil.
16. Juniper.

17. Kava Kava.

18. Licorice.

19. Marjoram essential oil.

20. Meadow saffron.

21. Mugwort essential oil.

22. Myrrh essential oil.

23. Pennyroyal, including essential oil.

24. Poke root.

25. Rue.

26. Sage, including essential oil.

27. St. John's wort.

28. Senna.

29. Tansy.

30. Thyme essential oil.

31. White Peony.

32. Wintergreen essential oil.

33. Wormwood.

34. Yarrow.

35. Yellow dock.

36. Vitamin A.

3). Is there an easy way to know if a medication is safe to use during pregnancy?

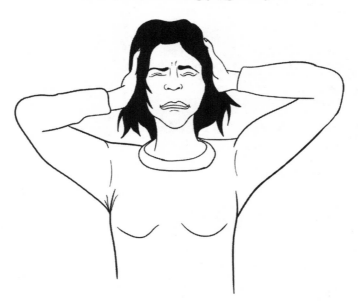

How to Determine If a Medication is Safe for Use During Pregnancy?

The US FDA (Food and Drug Administration) categorizes medications based upon their safety for using during both pregnancy and breastfeeding. For decades, the FDA used a letter based categorization to define medications as definitely safe, probably safe, unknown, probably unsafe, and definitely unsafe. In 2015, the FDA replaced the former letter based pregnancy risk categories with a new system with the goal of making the information presented more useful. While the new labeling improves the old format, it still does not provide a definitive "yes" or "no" answer in most cases, so clinical interpretation is still required on a case-by-case basis.

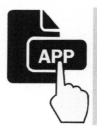

Curious if a medication is safe to use during pregnancy? Check out the FDA Medication Information feature of the app. Before you start any new medication, be sure to speak with your medical provider.

Before taking a new medication or continuing a pre-pregnancy medication, be sure to reach out to your provider first, and then check out the "FDA Medication Information" feature of the app.

4). How are medications classified for safety during pregnancy?

FDA Pregnancy Risk Categories before 2015 And After 2015?

In 1979, the FDA (the U.S Food and Drug Administration) established the A, B, C, D or X letter based risk classification system. These former pregnancy categories can still be found widely in package inserts, and they include:

1. **Category A:** These are the safest drugs to take during pregnancy as adequate and well-controlled studies have shown no fetal risk.

2. **Category B:** Animal reproduction studies have shown no risks when these medications were used during pregnancy. Class B medications are considered safe to take during pregnancy.

3. **Category C:** These medications have not been researched enough to determine if they are safe for use during pregnancy. Potential benefits may warrant use of the drug in pregnant women despite potential risks, but this risk-benefit ratio has to be examined by patient and provider.

4. **Category D:** Use of these medications has been shown to cause adverse reactions in humans. In serious or life-threatening conditions, potential benefits may still warrant use of the drug during pregnancy, but once again, the risk-benefit ratio has to be examined by the patient and provider.

5. **Category X:** A pregnant woman should NEVER use these drugs. Studies in animals or humans have demonstrated definitive evidence of human fetal risk. Regardless of potential

benefits of use, the risks involved in pregnant women clearly outweigh the potential benefits.

For years the FDA received complaints that the A/B/C/D/X categories did not provide patients or clinicians with all of the necessary information to make medication decisions during pregnancy. In 2015, the FDA devised a new labeling system that it says is designed to equip patients and clinicians better to make responsible medication decisions during pregnancy. **The Pregnancy and Lactation Labeling Rule (PLLR)** went into effect on June 30, 2015, but its use will be phased in over time based upon when a medication received initial FDA approval. Medications approved for use before June 2001 are not subject to the PLLR rule at all. The A, B, C, D and X risk categories, in use since 1979, have now replaced with narrative sections and subsections to include:

1. **Pregnancy** (includes Labor and Delivery):
   - Pregnancy Exposure Registry: Information about how to access and contribute to a registry monitoring use and outcomes during pregnancy.
   - Risk Summary: Summarize all of the possible risks of use.
   - Clinical Considerations: What risks and benefits of use need to be considered.
   - Data: Risk data accumulated thus far.

2. **Lactation** (includes Nursing Mothers)
   - Risk Summary.
   - Clinical Considerations.
   - Data.

3. **Females and Males of Reproductive Potential**
   - Pregnancy Testing.
   - Contraception.
   - Infertility.

CHAPTER 25

CREATING A BIRTH PLAN

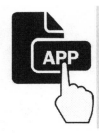

Don't forget to download the Everything Pregnancy app!

1). Okay, what exactly is a birth plan?

Should I create a birth plan and what is a birth plan anyway?

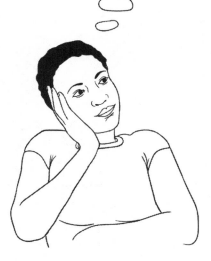

The Birth Plan: What is it and Why is it Important?

What is a Birth Plan?

A Birthing Plan is a simple, concise, written statement detailing what you and your partner would and would not like during the labor and delivery process. The Birth Plan generally covers things from induction of labor, pain control, and extent of fetal monitoring during labor to who cuts the umbilical cord after delivery and whether or not to give your baby vaccinations. Like most other things labor and delivery related, a birth plan is highly individualized. Just remember that life happens, and sometimes despite the best-laid plans, things just don't go as we envision they might. So, have a plan, know what you want and share that, but be flexible and realize that in the interest of your safety and the safety of your little bundle of joy, sometimes not every part of the Birth Plan may come to fruition.

Who Should I Share My Birth Plan with and When?

When it comes to the timing of sharing your Birth Plan, the sooner, the better. Generally, providers will be amenable to most Birth Plan requests as long as they don't endanger the safety of mother or baby. You don't, however, want to catch your provider or the hospital/birthing center staff off guard by presenting the plan for the first time when you are in labor, especially if your plan is detailed. We, therefore, recommend sharing your birth plan with your provider as soon as possible and definitely by the time you are entering the third trimester. Your provider will usually include a copy of the birth plan in your chart and make sure that the hospital or birthing center receives a copy as well. Nevertheless, it is always a good idea to have a few copies with you when you go into labor.

TO DO LIST

Start working on your Birth Plan as soon as possible and try to have it finished by the start of the third trimester so that you can share it with your medical provider.

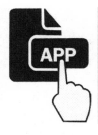

The Getting Ready for Delivery section of the app has a complete Birth Plan template that you can use to create and share your birth plan.

2). Okay, So How Do I Make a Birth Plan?

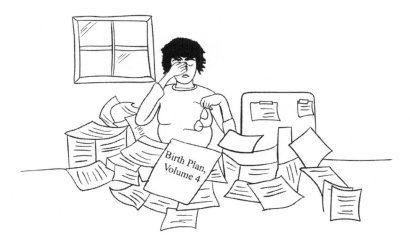

Birth Plan, Volume 4

Creating Your Birth Plan:

Now you know that the Twin Docs have you covered. Here is everything that you need to devise your very own Birth Plan:

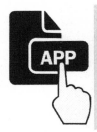

The Getting Ready for Delivery section of the app has a complete Birth Plan template that you can use to create and share your birth plan.

Opening: Opening: The opening is just a nice way to introduce yourself and your partner to the people who will be caring for your family in the hospital or birthing center. A good birth plan template follows, but of course, feel free to make the changes or additions that work best for you.

From: [*Insert your names here*]

Dear Caregivers and staff at [Insert name of Your Chosen Hospital or Birthing Center]*, we have chosen your outstanding facility to welcome our new bundle of joy, and we are requesting your assistance in helping us realize our goal of a healthy and happy birth experience. We educated ourselves before making our Birth Plan and feel that we are prepared to follow through on the points listed. We understand that complications do arise and in such instances, we fully trust our caregivers to make the necessary decisions. We simply ask that things be explained to us as the process moves along and that time permitting, we are allowed to have a private conversation between mother and partner after an informed discussion with our care team. We greatly appreciate your cooperation in realizing our plan.*

Brief Statement of Pertinent Medical History: Certain aspects of your medical history are important for your caregivers to know and a quick re-statement of these items (because they should also be included in the medical records from your provider's office) is an excellent reminder for all involved in your care.

- ☐ *We are planning to bank our cord blood.*
- ☐ *I have Group B Strep.*
- ☐ *I am Rh-Negative.*
- ☐ *I have been diagnosed with Genital Herpes.*
- ☐ *I have been diagnosed with Gestational Diabetes.*
- ☐ *Other pertinent medical history: _____.*
- ☐ *None of the above apply to me.*

If Labor Induction is Necessary: For a variety of reasons, induction of labor may be necessary. There are, however, a ton of options when it comes to inducing labor and many Birth Plans will state your preference when it comes to these options should it be necessary:

If my provider believes that induction is required, I would prefer the following method(s);

- ☐ *A cervical ripening vaginal insert (Cervidil) if my cervix is not ready for labor.*

- ☐ *A pill that is inserted into the vagina (Cytotec) if my cervix is not ready for labor. While widely and safely used for this purpose, Cytotec is not FDA approved for use during pregnancy.*

- ☐ *A cervical catheter to dilate and thin out my cervix if it is not yet ready for labor.*

- ☐ *Nipple stimulation or breast pumping to help me produce my own Oxytocin.*

- ☐ *IV Oxytocin to stimulate contractions if the cervix is ready for labor.*

- ☐ *Membrane stripping/sweeping to stimulate contractions.*

- ☐ *Other options: _____.*

My Desired Environment: This is a very important part of your Birth Plan because it lets everyone know in what type of environment you would like to labor and deliver your baby. Again, feel free to add anything that is not included here.

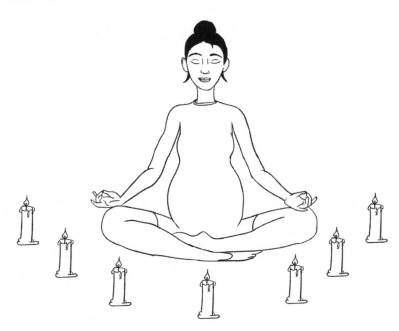

- ☐ *I would like the following people to be present while I labor:* [Insert your names here]
- ☐ *I would like the following people to be present when I deliver:* [Insert your names here]
- ☐ *I Am –OR- I Am Not Okay with students or other trainees being present*
- ☐ *I would like to bring and listen to music while I labor and deliver.*
- ☐ *I would like the lights to be as dim as possible.*
- ☐ *I would like to keep un-necessary discussion to a minimum in my room.*
- ☐ *I would like to use aromatherapy from home.*
- ☐ *I would like to have* [Insert your names here] *present for photos and video.*
- ☐ *I have personal comfort items that I would like to bring including: _____*
- ☐ *Other requests/desires: _____*

Pain Control During Labor: Be sure to state specifically your desires for pain control during labor. Things to consider include:

- ☐ *Do not ask me if I would like pain medication. If I want it, I will ask.*
- ☐ *I would like to be able to ambulate for as long as possible.*
- ☐ *I would like to use the birthing ball when possible.*
- ☐ *I would like to be able to take a shower or sit in the tub.*
- ☐ *I would like to have a massage.*
- ☐ *I would like to have acupuncture/acupressure.*
- ☐ *I would like to consider IV pain medications.*
- ☐ *I would like to consider an epidural.*

The First Stage of Labor: Remember, the first stage of labor is the fun part, starting with early or latent labor and continuing until your cervix is completely dilated and you're ready to push. Be sure to check out chapters 21 and 22 if you need a reminder about the different stages of labor and what to expect.

- ☐ *I would like to be allowed to labor at home as long as possible and if medically stable be allowed to return home if I am less than 5cm.*

- ☐ *I would like to be able to eat and drink as long as it is medically okay.*

- ☐ *I would like to avoid an IV if it is medically okay.*

- ☐ *If an IV is necessary, I would like a Heplock or Saline Lock (to protect the IV while allowing you to be mobile without an IV pole) placed.*

- ☐ *I would like intermittent fetal and uterine monitoring if medically okay.*

- ☐ *I would like my partner to remain with me throughout labor.*

- ☐ *I would like to minimize internal exams unless they are medically necessary.*

- ☐ *I only want internal monitors if medically necessary.*

- ☐ *I only want my bag of water broken if medically necessary.*

- ☐ *I will bring a gown or clothing from home and would prefer not to wear a hospital gown.*

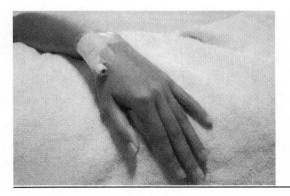 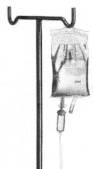

A saline lock or Heplock provides IV access if needed. An actual IV is connected only when IV fluids or IV medications are going to be given.

The Second Stage of Labor: The second stage of labor is when the rubber hits the road, starting when your cervix is completely dilated and ending when you hold your little bundle of joy for the first time.

- ☐ *I would rather risk a tear than have an episiotomy. I have done exercises at home to minimize the risk of tearing.*
- ☐ *I would like to choose the position that is most comfortable for me to push if medically stable.*
- ☐ *No stirrups, please.*
- ☐ *I would like to be allowed to view the delivery using a mirror.*
- ☐ *I would like to be allowed to touch my baby's head as she or he is crowning.*
- ☐ *Please don't coach me to push unless it is medically necessary. Let me push when my body tells me to push.*
- ☐ *I would like to avoid an operative vaginal delivery (vacuum or forceps) unless medically necessary.*
- ☐ *If an operative vaginal delivery is necessary, I prefer a vacuum as opposed to forceps.*
- ☐ *If an intervention is required, please explain everything to me.*
- ☐ *I would like the environment to be as quiet as possible during my delivery.*
- ☐ *I do not want the cord to be clamped or cut until it has stopped pulsating.*
- ☐ *I would like my partner to cut the umbilical cord.*
- ☐ *If my baby is stable, I want her or him placed directly on my abdomen or chest immediately after delivery.*
- ☐ *Please let my placenta deliver without traction or medication.*
- ☐ *I would like to breastfeed immediately.*
- ☐ *If stitching is necessary, please use local anesthesia to prevent discomfort.*

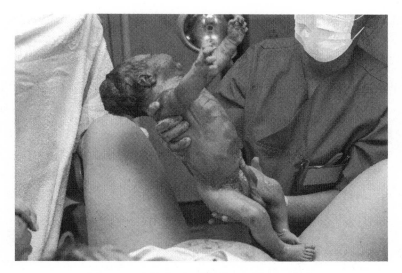

*Ask your medical provider if you can touch the
baby's head as she or he is crowning!*

The Third Stage of Labor: The third stage of labor starts after your baby
delivers and ends once the placenta delivers.

- ☐ *We would like our baby to remain with us at all times if medically
   able.*

- ☐ *Please do not give vaccines without our permission.*

- ☐ *Please do not bathe our baby for the first 24 hours.*

- ☐ *Please bathe our baby as soon as possible.*

- ☐ *No pictures of our baby without our permission.*

- ☐ *I want to breastfeed right away.*

- ☐ *No bottles, please.*

- ☐ *Breast only. No pacifiers, artificial nipples, etc....*

- ☐ *Please perform all physical exams and assessments in the room
   with us.*

- ☐ *If the baby needs to leave the room, we would like my partner
   to be with her or him at all times.*

- ☐ *If the baby needs warming, we would like him or her to be
   placed on mother's abdomen with a blanket if medically able.*

If A Cesarean Section Becomes Necessary: Sometimes, a Cesarean section is necessary for the well-being of the mother or baby. If you need to deliver via C/Section, you still have options, and having a Birth Plan is still important.

☐ *If at all possible, we would like to avoid a Cesarean Delivery.*

☐ *If a C/Section is necessary, I would like my partner to be with me at all times.*

☐ *If at all possible, I would like to be conscious during the procedure.*

☐ *I would like to have immediate skin-to-skin contact with my baby in the Operating Room.*

☐ *If a C/Section is necessary, I would like to have a sheer drape so that I can see the birth of my baby.*

☐ *I would like to breastfeed as soon as possible and in the OR if feasible.*

☐ *I would like music to be playing if possible.*

My Placenta: If you have plans for your placenta after delivery, it is important to include these in your Birth Plan.

☐ *The hospital may dispose of my placenta in the usual manner.*

☐ *I would like to take my placenta home.*

☐ *I would like my placenta to be prepared for encapsulation.*

☐ *I would like my placenta to be banked with the following company:* [Insert your name here]_____.

Closing: Most people include a closing remark in their Birth Plan thanking the staff for their attention and adherence to your wishes.

We thank you in advance for your support and kind attention to our choices. We look forward to a beautiful birth.

_____

Father

_____

Mother

_____

Physician

Index

Index

Index

Index

Index

Index

Index

Index

Index

S

T

Index

Y

Yeast, 162, 167, 169, 178–179, 397
YOGA, 143, 230, 323

Z

Zantac, 109, 396
Zoloft, 294